Understanding Cancer Therapies

Understanding Health and Sickness Series
Miriam Bloom, Ph.D.
General Editor

Understanding Cancer Therapies

Helen S. L. Chan, M.B.B.S.,
F.R.C.P.(C), F.A.A.P

University Press of Mississippi
Jackson

www.upress.state.ms.us

The University Press of Mississippi is a member of the Association of American University Presses.

Copyright © 2007 by University Press of Mississippi
All rights reserved
Manufactured in the United States of America

First edition 2007

∞

Library of Congress Cataloging-in-Publication Data

Chan, Helen S. L.
   Understanding cancer therapies / Helen S. L. Chan. — 1st ed.
      p. cm. — (Understanding health and sickness series)
   Includes index.
   ISBN 1-57806-688-3 (cloth : alk. paper) — ISBN 1-57806-689-1
(pbk. : alk. paper) 1. Cancer—Treatment—Popular works. I. Title.
   RC263.C424 2006
   616.99'406—dc22

                                                            2006027622

British Library Cataloging-in-Publication Data available

Contents

Introduction

The goal of this book is to explain cancer therapies in terms
of their underlying principles and the biology of normal cells and
cancer cells that forms the basis of treatment. Cell biology is how
normal cells behave and how the body controls different aspects
of their existence; cancer biology is how cancer cells behave in
the body and respond to therapy. The overview in chapter 1
explains the current approach of combining different types of
treatment to improve the odds of curing a cancer, known as the
multidisciplinary management of cancer. Each subsequent chapter focuses on a type of treatment: basic treatments including
surgery, radiation, and chemotherapy; newer treatments known
as biologic therapies, including immunotherapy and hormonal
therapy; and the related areas bone marrow transplant, supportive therapy, alternative therapy, and palliative therapy. Many
promising novel therapies, some already in use and others still in
the developmental stage, are discussed in the chapter on the
search for cures: molecular targeted therapy, gene therapy, differentiating therapy, antiangiogenic therapy, antimetastatic therapy,
multidrug resistance reversal therapy, and preventive therapy.

Conventional terminology for cell biology and cancer biology and treatment will be used in this book. Genes, by con-
vention, are shown in italics. Human genes are in upper case
(e.g., *RAS* oncogene) and animal genes in lower case (e.g., *ras*
oncogene), while the proteins that they make are not in italics
(e.g., RAS protein). Chemotherapy brand names are shown
with the first letter capitalized (e.g., Cytoxan). Chemical
names are in lower case (e.g., cyclophosphamide), while standard abbreviations are in capitals (e.g., CPM).

Understanding Cancer Therapies

1. Overview on Cancer Therapies

Cancer is a dreaded disease, but many cancers can now be cured because of improvements in treatment. They include leukemia, lymphoma, soft tissue and bone sarcoma, and germ cell tumor in children and adults, as well as Wilms tumor and retinoblastoma in children. For cancers that still cannot be cured, patients are now living longer because of better care. For cancers that cannot be completely removed by surgery or destroyed by chemotherapy and radiotherapy, patients may be made more comfortable with palliative care. It now can be truly said of cancer therapies, "to cure sometimes, to relieve often, to comfort always." The present approach is to combine different types of treatment to improve the cure of cancer. This is known as the multidisciplinary management of cancer.

Surgery

The Approach.   Surgery is removal of cancer from the body, localized therapy effective only for cancers that have not spread to other parts of the body and that can be removed completely. Surgery has the advantage of removing both dividing and nondividing cancer cells and those sensitive or resistant to chemotherapy and radiation. Its use dates as far back as 1600 BC, when it was mentioned in an Egyptian papyrus from the Middle Kingdom. Modern cancer surgery started in 1809, when Ephraim MacDowell removed a huge ovarian tumor. More aggressive cancer surgery was possible after William Morton and Crawford Long introduced ether as anesthesia in 1846 and Joseph Lister introduced antiseptic techniques in 1867. Cancer surgeons now work in cancer centers and take part in clinical trials organized by surgical oncology cooperative groups, federally funded groups consisting of many centers that together investigate new treatments. Surgeons take a biopsy of the cancer so that the pathologist can confirm the diagnosis; remove the entire cancer and surrounding involved tissues after chemotherapy and radiation have shrunk the cancer; and do preventive surgery for certain conditions recognized to have a high risk of evolving into cancers.

Radiation

The Approach.   Radiotherapy uses x-rays or radioactivity from radioisotopes to stop the growth of cancers by reducing the rate of cell division (mitosis) or by damaging DNA synthesis in cancer cells. This localized therapy is only effective if the cancers have not spread to other parts of the body. Radiation works best for dividing cancer cells, and is usually ineffective against nondividing cancer cells. Its use dates from the pioneering work by Pierre and Marie Curie in the late nineteenth century. Basic knowledge of radiation physics, biology of tumor cells and normal cells, and the clinical approach to treatment are important for the understanding of radiation for cancers. These concepts will be discussed in the chapter on radiation.

Chemotherapy

The Approach.   Chemotherapy, the use of drugs and chemicals to selectively destroy cancer cells, is systemic therapy that treats both the cancer and cells that have spread throughout the body. It works best for dividing cancer cells and is usually ineffective against nondividing cancer cells. In the past, chemotherapy was looked on as poison because the drugs were unreliable and toxic. Modern chemotherapy, dating from 1950–1960, is now effective, and selective in destroying more cancer cells than normal cells—the result of better understanding the biology of cancers, development of specific agents, experience with chemotherapy combinations, and advances in supportive therapy. Modern treatment can cure many cancers using combination chemotherapy in safe dosages, by safe administration, according to safe schedules, and with appropriate supportive therapies, as discussed in chapter 3. In cancer centers, a multidisciplinary team approach is generally used to provide total care for patients. Tumor Boards are held to review findings and assign appropriate protocols or clinical trial treatments. Patient and family conferences allow open communication and discussion of treatment options, so that there is full informed consent for treatment.

Biologic Therapy

The Approach.   Biologic therapy includes immunotherapy (manipulation of the immune response to treat cancer) and hormonal therapy (use of mammalian substances for therapy). Biologic therapy is systemic therapy that treats both the cancer and cells that have spread throughout the body, and works on both dividing and nondividing cancer cells. Related fields include bone marrow transplant, supportive therapy, alternative therapy, and palliative therapy.

Immunotherapy.   This is activation of the immune system to recognize and kill cancer cells. Immunotherapy is most useful for treating certain cancers, such as kidney cancer, that do not respond to chemotherapy. The immune system of the body recognizes "self" from "nonself"; it tolerates self but reacts against and eliminates nonself. Immunotherapy works by making cancer cells look more like nonself and boosting the immune response to kill them. The immune system works through body cells (cellular components) or body fluids (humoral components). Cellular components include blood cells such as lymphocytes, monocytes, macrophages, basophils, and eosinophils; support cells such as antigen-presenting dendritic cells and blood vessel endothelial cells; and tissue cells from the thymus, lymph nodes, and bone marrow. Humoral components include proteins called cytokines and antibodies. Cytokines include interferons and interleukins, naturally occurring, hormonelike substances that regulate the immune system. Antibodies are proteins that can find and kill cancer cells directly or activate the immune system to attack cancer cells. Synthetic cancer vaccines made from a patient's own cancer cells may be used to stimulate the body to recognize and kill those cancer cells.

Hormonal Therapy.   Hormones are natural secretions of the body that stimulate the growth of hormone-sensitive tissues, such as the breast, uterus, and prostate gland. When cancers arise in these organs, their growth and spread may be promoted by the body's own hormones. These hormone-dependent cancers have receptors, structures that recognize specific hormones. These cancers may be treated with drugs that block hormone production or change the way hormones work, and by removing organs, such as the ovaries or testes, that secrete hormones. Antihormones, or hormones with opposite functions, are agents that can block hormone production or change the way hormones work. Hormones may also treat some symptoms of cancer, such as poor appetite and emaciation.

Bone Marrow Transplant. Nowadays this includes collecting stem cells from the bone marrow or peripheral blood. Stem cells are nonspecialized cells that can replicate themselves. Stem cells can be given back to the patient as rescue after very-high-dose chemotherapy and/or radiation to the whole body, treatments not normally possible because they will kill the patient by destroying the bone marrow. The supralethal treatment is called the conditioning regimen, chosen for mainly marrow toxicity, rather than organ toxicity for which there is no rescue. Given like a blood transfusion, stem cells find their way into the bone marrow, to reproduce and repopulate it in a few weeks. A transplant may be from the patient's own stem cells (autologous) or from closely matched stem cells from other people (allogeneic).

Supportive Therapy. These therapies support the well-being of patients so that they can tolerate chemotherapy and radiation. Examples include blood transfusion for anemia and platelet transfusion for low platelet count or bleeding. Since cancer therapy can continue only as long as patients tolerate the treatment, supportive therapy may make the difference between cure and failure to cure the cancer. Open discussion of potential complications, counseling, and providing supportive therapy ensure that patients enjoy a better quality of life during treatment.

Alternative and Complementary Therapy. Alternative and complementary therapy describe treatments practiced outside conventional Western medicine. Alternative therapy is used instead of conventional therapy, while complementary therapy is used to supplement conventional therapy. Both consist of healing philosophies and practices not currently accepted therapy because they have not been tested in clinical trials or have been shown to be ineffective on testing. Both focus on promoting well-being, treating symptoms, improving general health, and stimulating the immune system. Many patients turn to alternative therapy after conventional medicine has nothing more to offer, or because they believe that the risks of conventional treatment outweigh the risks of alternative therapy. Since it is reported that up to 70 percent of patients use complementary or alternative therapy, it is important to make sure that they do not cause complications or interfere with conventional therapy.

Palliative Therapy.   The purpose of palliative therapy is to provide a good quality of life for patients when surgery is no longer possible and chemotherapy and radiation have failed to cure their cancers. The goal is to provide the best possible care in the home or hospice and prolong the valuable time that dying patients have for spending with their families. The guiding principle is to avoid aggressive measures that cause pain and complications. The emphasis is to provide comfort measures.

Novel Therapies

The Approach.   Novel therapies—new therapies already in use or promising therapies still in the research stage—include molecular therapy, gene therapy, differentiating therapy, antiangiogenic therapy, antimetastatic therapy, drug resistance reversal therapy, and preventive therapy.

Molecular Targeted Therapy.   Molecular therapy attacks how body cells sense their environment and communicate with each other, using what are known as signaling pathways. Signaling pathways regulate all aspects of the normal lives and functions of cells, including their replication, maturation (differentiation), repair of damages, aging (senescence), and the program that destroys damaged or aging cells (apoptosis). Signals are transmitted by ligands, which are secreted by cells. Receptors are structures on cells that detect ligand signals. Ligands bind to receptors to set off a cascade of secondary activities. These include proteins binding to other proteins forming complexes with specific functions. Small molecules are produced to act as second messengers to further spread the signals. Additional pathways are triggered that cooperate with or counteract the original action, providing the checks and balances for the system. Some signaling pathways are defective in cancer cells, so they escape from programs that regulate the activities of normal cells. Molecular targeted therapy is designed to attack these defective pathways unique to cancer cells but absent in normal cells, blocking vital activities like growth or essential sites like receptors. Molecular targeted therapy is still experimental.

Gene Therapy. For gene therapy, modified DNA from viruses may be put into target genes to kill cancer cells that are susceptible because of their genetic pattern. Alternatively, a special DNA sequence may be put into target genes to activate a death signal that stops cancer cells from replicating. These target genes are then inserted into cancer cells by using a carrier called a vector, which is usually one of the RNA retroviruses. Gene therapy is still experimental. It has great future potential but many clinical limitations at present. It is difficult to introduce enough target genes into cancer cells, and have the target genes function effectively in killing cancer cells.

Differentiating Therapy. Cancer cells retain the ability to replicate relentlessly because they have not become mature and specialized. Drugs causing differentiation may stop this endless cell division. Vitamin A derivatives, such as retinoids, and some forms of vitamin D have differentiating properties and can suppress cell division and prevent the start of cancers (carcinogenesis). Differentiating therapy is still experimental.

Antiangiogenic Therapy. Antiangiogenic therapy destroys the blood supply to cancers, starving them of nutrients and oxygen that are essential for growth. Cancers make their own proangiogenic factors to promote the growth of tumor blood vessels, which are counteracted by antiangiogenic factors produced by immune cells that infiltrate cancers. Proangiogenic and antiangiogenic factors bind to receptors on the endothelial cells that make up blood vessels. The balance between proangiogenic and antiangiogenic factors regulates the survival or death of endothelial cells and the formation of capillaries (small blood vessels). These factors also control the processes by which cancer cells metastasize, their migration, invasion through blood vessel walls, and spreading into other organs. Antiangiogenic therapy interferes with these processes. This therapy is still experimental. It is not toxic, does not become resistant, works on both dividing and nondividing cancer cells, and treats both the cancer and cells that have spread throughout the body. However, it has to be used for years and is ineffective against large, untreated cancers.

Antimetastatic Therapy. Cancer cells migrate, invade, and metastasize in a complex way, synchronized by a number of signaling pathways. Migration is regulated by integrin signals. Integrins are cell surface molecules that can sense the environment and signal cancer cells to move and to stick to and invade through capillary walls. Cancer cells sticking to capillary walls or to each other are regulated by cadherin and CD44 signals. Cadherins are another type of cell surface molecules; CD44 is a cell membrane glycoprotein. Invasion by cancer cells into small blood vessels is mediated by the metalloproteinase enzymes, which dissolve different proteins forming blood vessel walls. Whether or not the clumps of tumor cells take root and grow into metastases depends on the tissue environment, and the acquisition of a tumor blood supply. Antimetastatic therapy is the experimental use of inhibitors of integrins, cadherins, CD44, and metalloproteinases to prevent cancer cells from migrating, invading, and metastasizing.

Drug Resistance Reversal Therapy. Drug resistance mechanisms are ways by which cancer cells avoid the toxic effects of chemotherapy. Cancer cells acquire drug resistance through mutations (genetic mistakes). Certain preexisting pathways have been preserved through evolution to protect normal cells from toxic substances in the environment. Mutations in these protective pathways allow cancer cells to avoid the toxic effects of chemotherapy. Mutations include making multiple copies of the drug resistance genes (amplification) and increased production of drug resistance proteins. These resistant cancer cells respond poorly to chemotherapy, and grow instead of die on treatment, causing poor prognosis. Reversal therapy uses experimental drugs or methods that bypass drug resistance. One major problem is the increase in chemotherapy toxicity. The blocking of drug resistance in cancer cells unfortunately also blocks protective mechanisms for normal cells. This is because the drug resistance mechanisms amplified in cancer cells are actually natural defense methods for normal cells.

Preventive Therapy. This is the use of nontoxic natural products or dietary supplements to prevent cancer formation. Preventive therapy sounds attractive but has limitations: it

cannot be used to cure established cancers, and may only prevent cancers recurring or secondary cancers developing as a
result of radiation. Preventive therapy is used mainly for
lesions that may evolve into cancers (premalignant), or for
cancers of the head and neck, lung, skin, cervix, breast, and
bladder. Preventive therapy is thought to work by causing
cells to mature and become specialized or by protecting cells
from compounds that cause cancer (carcinogens) by using
drugs that detoxify carcinogens (antioxidants). Agents with
differentiating properties include derivatives of vitamin A
such as retinoids and carotenoids, micronutrients such as selenium, multivitamins such as vitamins E and C, and other
compounds such as phytoestrogens, organosulfur, and protease inhibitors. Many of these agents occur naturally in vegetables, fruits, beans, and nuts.

Cancer Treatment and Results

Treatment Phases.   Cancer therapy is divided into phases,
blocks of treatment with a specific purpose. *Induction* is the
initial treatment to reduce the tumor load in the body.
Maintenance is continued therapy to kill the rest of the cancer
cells. *Reinduction* is more intensive therapy given periodically
to kill more cancer cells. *Intensification* is higher dose
chemotherapy to kill even more cancer cells, and may be
given with stem cell rescue for the bone marrow. *Central
nervous system prophylaxis* is therapy to prevent cancer or
leukemia cells spreading into the cerebrospinal fluid, where
systemic chemotherapy has difficulty entering. It may be
given by lumbar puncture (intrathecal therapy); or through
an Ommaya reservoir connected to the ventricular system
of the brain, as high-dose chemotherapy to better penetrate

into the cerebrospinal fluid; or by radiating the brain and spine. *Adjuvant chemotherapy* is given after surgery or radiation. *Neoadjuvant chemotherapy* is given before surgery or radiation. *Palliative chemotherapy* is given to relieve symptoms and pain or to prolong survival when there is no hope of cure.

Treatment Responses and Results. Response to treatment may be assessed as the response rate (percentage of treated responding to therapy), remission rate (percentage of treated achieving complete remission with no evidence of tumor), or control rate (percentage of treated with stabilization of disease). Short-term results of treatment may be assessed as complete response (no evidence of tumor), very good partial response (more than 90 percent of tumor gone), partial response (more than 50 percent of tumor gone), minor response (less than 10 percent of tumor gone), stable disease (no progression for at least one month), or progressive disease (no response). Long-term results of treatment may be assessed as cure rate (percentage of treated without relapse at five years from diagnosis), event-free rate (percentage of treated with no adverse events, such as relapse or death from any causes, at five years), and survival rate (percentage of treated alive, whether or not in remission, at five years). Generally, these results are quoted with the median follow-up, which is the observation time that has been reached by half of the patients.

The Prospect of Cure

The twelve most common childhood cancers are described in chapter 7. Cure rates for each cancer depend on whether the pathology is good or poor, the stage or extent of disease, surgical removal, response to chemotherapy and radiation, and whether there are good or poor biologic factors. Cure rates may be given as a range or as an overall figure. The low end of the range of cure rates represents metastatic, unfavorable, unresectable, or unresponsive disease, and the high end, localized, favorable, resectable, or responsive disease. Briefly, the overall cure rates are: leukemia (50–80 percent), brain and spinal cord tumors (20–90 percent), lymphoma (80 percent), neuroblastoma (20–100 percent), soft tissue sarcoma (60 percent), Wilms tumor (80 percent), bone sarcoma (60 percent), retinoblastoma (70 percent), germ cell tumors (80 percent), hepatoblastoma (60 percent), and melanoma and carcinoma of the skin, thyroid gland, salivary gland, nasopharynx, colon, and pancreas (cure rates similar to adults).

The twenty-four most common cancers in adults are described in chapter 8. Cure rates also depend on the pathology, stage, surgical removal, response to chemotherapy and radiation, and other prognostic factors. Briefly, the overall cure rates are: skin carcinoma (90 percent), prostate carcinoma (90 percent), breast carcinoma (85 percent), lung carcinoma (14 percent), colon carcinoma (62 percent), uterine carcinoma (84 percent), lymphoma (51–80 percent), bladder carcinoma (81 percent), ovarian carcinoma (40 percent), malignant melanoma (88 percent), anorectal carcinoma (60 percent), oropharyngeal carcinoma (53 percent), leukemia (20–60 percent), renal cell carcinoma (60 percent), pancreatic carcinoma (4 percent), uterine cervix carcinoma (71 percent), stomach carcinoma (21 percent), central nervous system malignancies (31 percent), hepatocellular and biliary carcinoma (5 percent), multiple myeloma (29 percent), esophageal carcinoma (11 percent), soft tissue sarcoma (50 percent), testicular carcinoma (70 percent), and bone sarcoma (50 percent).

2. How Cancer Therapy Is Determined

Staging determines the extent of the cancer, and what the best therapy is. One staging schema is the TNM system, in which T stands for tumor, N for lymph nodes, and M for metastases. In a more generic staging schema, Stage I stands for localized, Stage II for regional, Stage III for extensive, and Stage IV for metastatic disease. Staging is determined by the history, physical examination, laboratory and radiologic tests, and biopsy of the cancer, lymph nodes and metastases.

History and Physical Examination

The general effects of a cancer are often due to release of cytokines, which are natural hormonelike substances that regulate the immune system. Tumor necrosis factor is one such cytokine that causes fever, night sweating, emaciation, poor appetite, weakness, anemia, low blood sugar, and high blood acidity. Other symptoms and signs are caused by the tumor mass and its compression of adjacent normal tissues. The cancer may present only as a painless lump, or as pain from compression of nerves, blood vessels, bone, and bone marrow. Sometimes the compression can cause an acute emergency, such as obstruction of the flow of cerebrospinal fluid, or compression of the spinal cord, airway, heart and its great vessels, bowel and urinary tract. Alternately, patients may present with paraneoplastic syndromes such as high uric acid, potassium, calcium, and phosphate released from the breakdown of leukemia or lymphoma cells, which block the urinary tract and cause kidney failure.

Blood, Urine and Other Examinations

Laboratory tests determine the general health of the patient and may confirm the diagnosis. General tests include the complete blood count (CBC), urine test (urinalysis), liver and renal function tests, and blood chemistry. Specific tests include biologic, hormonal, enzyme, or genetic tumor markers (table 2.1), which determine the diagnosis and predict prognosis, response to therapy, recurrence, and tumor progression. Some tests may be useful as mass screening tools for certain cancers.

Radiologic and Imaging Studies

Besides helping to make the diagnosis, these tests determine prognosis, response to therapy, tumor recurrence, progression, and metastases.

X-rays. X-rays, used for screening purposes, are back-to-front or side-to-side views of the body.

Computed Axial Tomography (CT). CT scans consist of multiple cross-sectional x-rays of the body, which the computer reconstructs into side-to-side and top-to-bottom views. They give detailed pictures of tumors that can be intensified with injected or ingested dyes. Tumors are distinguished from normal tissues by their texture, density, and blood supply. CT pictures can now be enhanced by real-time imaging, multiphase imaging, multidetector scanning, and virtual reality displays.

Table 2.1 Summary of Cancer-Related Markers for Diagnosis and Prognosis

Classes	Markers	Source	Applicable diseases
Tumor-specific markers	leukemia cells	blood and cerebrospinal fluid	acute and chronic lymphoid or myeloid leukemia and lymphoma
	cancer cells	sputum	lung cancer
	cancer cells	urine	bladder and renal-cell cancers, Wilms tumor
	cancer cells in PAP (Papanicolaou) smear	mucus from the cervix	cervix cancer
	prostate-specific antigen (PSA) and prostate-specific membrane antigen (PSMA)	blood	prostate cancer
	carcinoembrionic antigen (CEA) and CA 19-9	blood	stomach, gallbladder, and colorectal cancers
	CA-125	blood	ovarian, stomach, and endometrial cancers
	α-fetoprotein	blood	germ cell and liver cancer
	β-human chorionic gonadotrophin	blood	germ cell, testicular, ovarian, and trophoblastic malignancy, choriocarcinoma and liver cancer
	alkaline phosphatase	blood	osteosarcoma

(Continued)

Table 2.1 (*Continued*)

Classes	Markers	Source	Applicable diseases
	β$_2$-microglobulin, C-reactive protein	blood	multiple myeloma
	Bence Jones protein (immunoglobulin light chains)	urine	
	serotonin and its breakdown product, 5-hydroxyindolacetic acid	blood and urine	carcinoid tumor
	vanillylmandelic acid (VMA), homovanillic acid (HVA), and their breakdown products: epinephrine, norepinephrine, metanephrine, and dopamine	urine	neuroblastoma, pheochromocytoma
Genetic markers	*BRCA1, BRCA2* gene mutations	blood	breast and ovarian cancers
	RB1 gene mutations	blood	retinoblastoma, bone and soft tissue sarcomas
	mismatch repair gene mutations	blood	colon, bowel, uterus, and other hereditary nonpolyposis colorectal (HNPCC) cancers
	microsatellite instability	blood	
	APC gene mutations	blood	colon and bowel cancers

Hormonal markers	somatostatin	blood	carcinoid tumor, neuroblastoma, pancreatic and small cell lung cancer, lymphoma, meningioma
	parathyroid hormone and high blood calcium	blood	parathyroid cancer
	cortisol, aldosterone, and their breakdown products	blood	adrenal cancer
Enzyme markers	lactic dehydrogenase	blood	leukemia and lymphoma
Nonspecific markers	ferritin	blood	neuroblastoma
	erythrocyte sedimentary rate (ESR)blood	blood	leukemia and lymphoma
		feces	colon cancer

Magnetic Resonance Imaging (MRI). MRI also consists of multiple cross-sectional views of the body, which the computer reconstructs into side-to-side, top-to-bottom and whole-body views. The machine contains a large magnet that changes the spinning of hydrogen nuclei, lining them up along the magnetic field. A radiofrequency pulse, of the same frequency as the hydrogen nuclei, is used to line up the hydrogen nuclei transverse to the direction of the magnetic field. When the radiofrequency pulse is stopped, the hydrogen nuclei relax back into their original alignment, sending out electromagnetic signals that the computer generates into images. There is no radiation exposure with MRI. It is even better than CT at imaging tumors, and the pictures can be enhanced with injected rare earth metals like gadolinium. It shows details of arteries, veins, lymphatics, and nerves, structures like bone, joint, brain and spinal cord, and hollow organs like bladder, cervix, uterus, and bone marrow space. However, it is a longer procedure that requires general anesthesia in young children. Also, it is not ideal for looking at structures containing air, such as the lungs.

Positron Emission Tomography (PET). PET scans detect with gamma cameras, the photon energy released from ^{11}carbon, ^{13}nitrogen, ^{15}oxygen or ^{18}fluorodeoxyglucose (^{18}F) radioisotopes. As the photon energy is absorbed, electrons rotating around the atomic nuclei are ejected, creating more photon energy that ejects other electrons. For example, cancer cells use more glucose than normal cells, which is detected by ^{18}F-PET. PET can distinguish live from dead tumors or scar tissues. However, PET cannot detect lesions smaller than 4 mm. Nor can it distinguish tumors from inflammatory tissues. PET results are difficult to interpret in low oxygen environments and after recent therapy. New markers are being developed to show differences between tumors and nontumors, such as amino acid and thymidine production or oxygen usage, or receptors for drugs, hormones, or drug resistance. PET combined with MRI is called functional MRI, which allows detection of smaller lesions.

Ultrasonography. Ultrasound and Doppler studies are used to provide a real-time map of the tumor and adjacent normal tissues, especially arteries and veins, direction of blood flow, and blood clots or tumor clumps within blood vessels.

Radionuclide Scans. Different radioisotopes are used to scan different organs to look for metastases. Bone scan uses a ^{99m}technicium compound to look for bone metastases or calcification within neuroblastoma. Liver scan uses a different ^{99m}technicium compound to look for lesions in the liver and spleen. Thyroid scan uses a third ^{99m}technicium compound or ^{123}I-sodium iodide to detect thyroid cancer and metastases. Gallium scan uses ^{67}Ga citrate to bind to transferrin receptors in sarcoma, lymphoma, melanoma, and lung and liver cancer. MIBG scan uses ^{131}I-metaiodobenzylguanidine to image neuroblastoma and pheochromocytoma. Some of these radioisotopes are also useful for cancer therapy, such as MIBG for neuroblastoma, or ^{131}I-sodium iodide for thyroid cancer.

Antibody and Peptide Imaging. Antibodies against tumor markers or their analogues (structurally similar compounds) may also be used to look for metastases. For example, ^{99m}technicium anti-CEA antibody is used to detect colorectal cancer metastases, ^{111}indium-labeled anti-PSMA antibody (ProstaScint) to detect prostate cancer metastases, and ^{111}indium-labeled pentetreotide (Octreoscan) to detect somatostatin receptors in carcinoid tumor, neuroblastoma and other cancers.

Other Imaging Studies. Some studies are used for baseline, ongoing and follow-up assessments of toxicity. Pulmonary function test assesses lung function in bleomycin and radiation therapy. Audiogram assesses hearing in cisplatin and carboplatin therapy. Echocardiogram and multigated angiography (MUGA scan) assess heart function in doxorubicin and daunorubicin therapy. Radioisotope glomerular filtration rate (GFR) assesses kidney function in cisplatin, carboplatin, and high-dose methotrexate therapy.

3. How Chemotherapy Works

Most children and many adults suffering from leukemia, lymphoma, soft tissue and bone sarcoma, and germ cell tumor can now be cured by chemotherapy. Most children with Wilms tumor, retinoblastoma, and hepatoblastoma also are cured with the help of chemotherapy. Even if chemotherapy is not curative, it can be used to relieve symptoms and prolong life when cancer has spread and cannot be removed by surgery or destroyed by radiotherapy. To understand how chemotherapy works it is important to understand cell biology as well as cancer biology. Cell biology is how normal cells behave and how the body controls different aspects of their existence. Cancer biology is how cancer cells behave in the body and respond to therapy. Essentially, cancer forms when the systems that regulate the activities of normal cells are disrupted. Cancer cells do not behave like normal cells, nor can they be kept in check by the same control mechanisms that regulate the behavior of normal cells.

Normal Cell Biology and Cancer Biology

How Cells Divide During the Cell Cycle.   All cells go through the cell cycle with the purpose of dividing. During the cell cycle, they make the deoxyribonucleic acid (DNA), ribonucleic acid (RNA), and proteins for duplicating the chromosomes and genes necessary for dividing into daughter cells. The cell cycle consists of several phases, each with a different purpose. The first phase is Gap 1 (G_1), in which RNA and proteins are made. The second phase is DNA synthesis (S). The third phase is Gap 2 (G_2), in which more RNA and proteins are made. The final phase, mitosis (M), is when each cell divides into two daughter cells. Daughter cells may continue dividing by "staying in cycle," or stop dividing and go into a resting phase (G_0). Alternatively, cells may stop dividing because they become mature and specialized in a process called differentiation, or age by undergoing senescence, or die in a program called apoptosis.

Genes That Control the Cell Cycle. Cyclin genes control cells moving from one phase of the cell cycle to another. These genes act as signals directing cells to make certain proteins and enzymes that are used to regulate cell division, differentiation, aging, or death. Enzymes that control the cell cycle, called the cyclin-dependent kinases or cdks, work with cyclin genes to control the activities of cells. This interaction between cyclin genes and cdk enzymes is inhibited by cdk inhibitors, which counterbalance the activity of cdk. Together, cyclin genes, cdks, and cdk inhibitors control how normal cells move through the cell cycle to achieve cell division. Cancer forms when this system is disrupted. Genes that can disrupt the cell cycle and promote cancer formation are called oncogenes. When oncogenes are switched on, they disrupt vital signaling pathways that control the cell cycle. Another type of genes, called tumor suppressor genes, causes cancer in a different way. Tumor suppressor genes promote cancer formation when switched off, causing loss of control of normal cellular functions and the body's ability to suppress tumor formation. Mistakes made by these genes when cells divide are called mutations. Certain mutations can cause cancer because they switch on oncogenes or switch off tumor suppressor genes.

How Mistakes Are Corrected at Cell Cycle Checkpoints.
Checkpoints are barriers that stop cells going through the cell cycle, so that mistakes made during DNA synthesis can be repaired. One example of an important checkpoint is between the G_1 phase (when RNA and proteins are made) and S phase (when DNA is synthesized). Normally, the G_1/S checkpoint is switched off, allowing cells in G_1 to enter S. This normal G_1/S checkpoint switch-off is mediated by cyclin genes interacting with cdk enzymes, which inactivates an important protein, the RB protein; the RB protein releases its partner, E2F, a transcription factor that signals DNA to make RNA and protein, thus allowing cells in G_1 to enter S. When the G_1/S checkpoint has to be switched on, cells in G_1 are stopped from entering S. Things that can switch on the G_1/S checkpoint include DNA damage, such as from chemotherapy or radiation. DNA damage signals the *p53* tumor suppressor gene to make p53 protein. This p53 protein then switches on the cdk inhibitors, which stop cdk enzymes from interacting with the cyclin genes. This in turn allows the RB protein to become activated. The activated RB protein then binds to its partner, E2F, which signals the RNA and protein production from DNA to stop, thus stopping cells in G_1 from entering S. This gives time for the DNA damage to be repaired. Other checkpoints, occurring at S and G_2/M, serve similar purposes.

How Cancer Forms and Progresses if Cell Cycle Checkpoints Do Not Work. Cancer forms when tumor suppressor genes are switched off by mutations, causing loss of control of normal cellular functions and the body's ability to suppress tumor formation. One important example is mutation of the *p53* tumor suppressor genes. When the *p53* gene is mutated in cancer cells, their cell cycle controls become defective, allowing them to divide without stopping or differentiating into mature, specialized cells. In effect, the cancer cells behave as if they are "immortal." In malignancies such as Burkitt lymphoma, the cancer cells also divide very fast, doubling their numbers within hours. Furthermore, the cancer cells do not age normally and die like normal cells, because their senescence and apoptosis pathways are defective. Nor do the cancer cells use the apoptosis program, like normal cells, to self-destruct when they acquire mutations or make irreparable mistakes. Additionally, cancers cells may have acquired mutations that cause resistance to chemotherapy or radiation.

How Chemotherapy Works at Different Points in The Cell Cycle.   Chemotherapy drugs are designed to work at different phases of the cell cycle. Most drugs work at the S phase, when DNA is synthesized, or the M phase, when mitosis occurs. Therefore, chemotherapy generally kills only dividing cancer cells. Fast-dividing cancers respond better to chemotherapy than slow-dividing ones. Small cancers respond better to chemotherapy than large ones, in which cell division has slowed down. Each chemotherapy treatment (called a cycle) kills a proportion of normal cells as well as cancer cells. Because of this, time must be allowed between treatment cycles for the normal cells to recover. During this recovery time, however, the cancer cells also recover in numbers. Therefore, chemotherapy is only effective if the normal cells recover faster than cancer cells. Chemotherapy is ineffective if the cancer cells recover faster than normal cells, growing back completely by the next treatment. It takes the cumulative result of multiple treatments, each killing a proportion of the cancer cells, to eradicate the entire tumor. Chemotherapy rarely kills nondividing cancer cells. Therefore, cancers with a high proportion of nondividing cancer cells are considered refractory to chemotherapy.

Chemotherapy Works in Different Phases of the Cell Cycle

During the cell cycle, most drugs kill only dividing cancer cells, as shown in Table 3.1. Most of these drugs also work only at a particular phase of the cell cycle. Only a few classes of drugs can work independent of the cell cycle by damaging DNA and killing dividing cancer cells. Even fewer drugs work in the G_0 resting phase to kill nondividing cancer cells.

Normal Functions of Cells Susceptible to Chemotherapy Damage

DNA Structure.   When James D. Watson and Francis Crick discovered the structure of DNA in 1953, their work led to finding how DNA is made (DNA replication), how DNA directs cells to make RNA (RNA transcription), and how RNA directs cells to make proteins (RNA translation). DNA is normally packaged into genes that make up chromosomes within the cell nucleus. DNA exists as two strands tightly wound together in a double helix. Each strand of DNA is a chain of nucleotides. Each nucleotide contains a deoxyribose sugar and a purine base (adenine or guanine) or a pyrimidine base (thymine or cytosine). Chemical bonds between the bases hold the two DNA strands together, with adenine (A) binding only to thymine (T), and guanine (G) only to cytosine (C), in a process called complementary base-pairing.

RNA is Another Site of Chemotherapy Damage.   RNA exists as a single strand of nucleotides. Each nucleotide in RNA contains a ribose sugar, rather than the deoxyribose sugar of DNA, and a purine base (adenine or guanine) or a pyrimidine

Table 3.1 Chemotherapy Drugs and where they Work in the Cell Cycle

Classes	Subclasses	Where they Work in the Cell Cycle	Drugs
Alkylating agents		cell cycle–independent	mechlorethamine (Mustargen), cyclophosphamide (Cytoxan), ifosfamide, melphalan, chlorambucil, thiotepa, mitomycin C, dibromodulcitol, busulfan, procarbazine, dacarbazine
Platinum compounds		cell cycle–independent	cisplatin, carboplatin, oxaliplatin
Cytotoxic antibiotics		cell cycle–independent	doxorubicin, daunorubicin, idarubicin, epirubicin, mitoxantrone, dactinomycin
Antimetabolites		S	methotrexate, cytarabine, gemcitabine, cladribine, fludarabine, 2-deoxycoformycin, 6-mercaptopurine, 6-thioguanine, 5-fluorouracil
Plant alkaloids	Vinca alkaloids	M	vincristine, vinblastine, vindesine
	Podophyllotoxins	G_2	etoposide, teniposide
	Camptothecins	G_2	camptothecin, irinotecan, topotecan
	Taxanes	G_2/M	paclitaxel, docetaxel
Miscellaneous agents		S	hydroxyurea
		G_2	bleomycin
		G_1	asparaginase, steroids (also work in S)
Nitrosoureas		cell cycle–independent	carmustine, lomustine (also work in G_0)

base (uracil or cytosine). In RNA, uracil (U) replaces thymine in the pyrimidine base.

How DNA Replicates. The double strand of DNA is first unwound to expose the nucleotides. The DNA polymerase enzyme then assembles nucleotides to make a new strand of DNA by using the complementary base-pairing process. The new DNA is synthesized based on an existing coding pattern (DNA template). For example, an ATTCAG sequence on the DNA template is matched by the complementary TAAGTC sequence in the new DNA made. The newly made DNA strands then rewind together forming two separate double helices.

How DNA Information is Transcribed into RNA. DNA information is passed into messenger RNA (mRNA). The RNA polymerase enzyme similarly assembles nucleotides to make RNA according to a DNA template, except that uracil replaces thymine during the complementary base-pairing process. For example, an ATTCAG sequence on the DNA template is matched by the complementary UAAGUC sequence in the new mRNA made.

How RNA Information is Translated into Proteins. Before mRNA leaves the nucleus to pass the DNA information to cells that make proteins, it has to be spliced. Splicing cuts out introns, intervening regions that provide no information, to leave exons that contain the coding information. Proteins are made in structures in the cells called ribosomes. Ribosomes contain ribosomal RNA (rRNA), which decodes the DNA information within mRNA, and transfer RNA (tRNA), which matches this information with the correct amino acids to make proteins. The DNA information exists as a *triplet code*. Each of the twenty existing amino acids is represented by a different triplet code. For example, the triplet code for the amino acid methionine is ATG, for threonine it is ACC, for serine TCC, and for phenylalanine TTC. Different types of proteins—such as enzymes, hormones and antibodies—are made up of chains of amino acids in different sequences. Hair, for instance, is made of the protein keratin, which starts with a methionine-threonine-serine-phenylalanine sequence. Proteins function only after they have acquired three-dimensional configurations by twisting their amino acid chains into ball-like structures. Proteins sometimes need to be modified further before they become active, such as by addition of a phosphate group (phosphorylation) or removal of a phosphate group (dephosphorylation).

Different Mechanisms by which Chemotherapy Damages Cells

There are six main classes of chemotherapy agents that can damage cancer cells in different ways:

- *Alkylating agents* make breaks in DNA, or link together DNA, stopping DNA synthesis and repair and RNA transcription.
- *Platinum compounds* combine with DNA, making breaks in DNA or linking together DNA.
- *Antimetabolites* substitute themselves for normal components of cells, stopping vital functions of cells, and making proteins and enzymes that cannot function properly.
- *Topoisomerase-interactive agents* inhibit the topoisomerase enzymes that the control the three-dimensional structure of DNA necessary for function.
- *Antimicrotubule agents* inhibit formation of the tubulin framework of the mitotic spindle that is essential for mitosis.
- *Miscellaneous agents* inhibit different critical processes in cells.

Alkylating Agents

Mechanisms of Action.   Alkylating agents are highly reactive compounds containing electron-rich nitrogen, sulfur, and oxygen atoms. A form of DNA damage called alkylation is caused by adding an alkyl group (R–CH–CH) or substituting an alkyl group for a hydrogen atom. This process makes breaks in DNA or links together the two DNA strands (interstrand cross-linkage) or parts of the same DNA strand (intrastrand cross-linkage). This interferes with DNA replication and repair and also prevents RNA transcription. Some alkylating agents, such as cyclophosphamide and ifosfamide, have to be activated by liver enzymes, while others, such as mechlorethamine, require no activation. Table 3.2 shows subclasses of alkylating agents, gives examples of the drugs, and summarizes their mechanisms of action and their use for treatment of different cancers.

Platinum Compounds

Mechanisms of Action.   These agents were developed when it was observed that bacteria and cells were killed in the electric field between platinum electrodes. Platinum compounds damage DNA by combining with it to form complexes, linking together the two DNA strands or parts of the same DNA strand. Platinum compounds contain a central platinum atom surrounded by chlorine and ammonia atoms. The parent drug, cisplatin, which has two ammonia atoms next to two chlorine atoms, can cause considerable kidney toxicity and hearing loss. A substitution of the two chlorine atoms produces carboplatin, which causes less kidney toxicity and less hearing loss. Another substitution produces oxaliplatin, which is toxic to nerves rather than to kidney and hearing. Table 3.3

Table 3.2 Mechanisms of Action and Diseases Treated by Alkylating Agents

Subclasses	Mechanisms of Action	Drugs	Diseases Treated
Nitrogen mustards	contain highly reactive aziridinium rings, making breaks in DNA or linking together double-strand DNA	mechlorethamine (Mustargen)	Hodgkin lymphoma
		cyclophosphamide (Cytoxan)	Hodgkin and non-Hodgkin lymphoma, brain and germ cell tumor, breast cancer, neuroblastoma, Ewing sarcoma, rhabdomyosarcoma, multiple myeloma
		ifosfamide	Ewing sarcoma, rhabdomyosarcoma, non-Hodgkin lymphoma, neuroblastoma, brain tumor
		melphalan	multiple myeloma, bone marrow transplant
		chlorambucil	chronic lymphocytic leukemia, non-Hodgkin and Hodgkin lymphoma, autoimmune disease
Aziridines	contain less reactive aziridine rings, making breaks in DNA or linking together DNA	thiotepa	bone marrow transplant
		mitomycin C	breast, esophagus, and gastrointestinal cancer
Epoxides	derived from nitrogen mustards but have epoxide groups	dibromodulcitol	brain tumor, breast and cervix cancer

Alkyl sulfonates	make breaks in DNA or link together double-strand DNA	busulfan (Myeleran)	chronic myelogenous leukemia, bone marrow transplant
Nitrosoureas	react with single-strand DNA and cross-link double-strand DNA	carmustine (BCNU) lomustine (CCNU)	brain tumor, multiple myeloma, bone marrow transplant
Hydrazines and triazines	work like nitrosoureas	procarbazine dacarbazine (DTIC)	Hodgkin lymphoma Hodgkin lymphoma, malignant melanoma
		temozolomide	malignant melanoma, brain tumor

Table 3.3 Mechanisms of Action and Diseases Treated by Platinum Compounds

Subclass	Mechanisms of Action	Drugs	Diseases Treated
Platinum compounds	(1) bind with DNA forming complexes	cisplatin	brain and germ cell tumor, neuroblastoma, hepatoblastoma, ovarian cancer; multiple myeloma
	(2) damage DNA to produce interstrand and intrastrand DNA cross-linkages	carboplatin	brain and germ cell tumor, neuroblastoma, hepatoblastoma, retinoblastoma, bone marrow transplant
		oxaliplatin	brain and germ cell tumor, neuroblastoma, hepatoblastoma

shows the platinum compounds, gives examples of the drugs, and summarizes their mechanisms of action and their use for treatment of different cancers.

Antimetabolites

Mechanism of Action. Metabolites are components of cells that they require for normal growth and metabolism. Antimetabolites are analogues of these metabolites. Analogues have structures similar to normal metabolites, so that when analogues are substituted for these metabolites, defective proteins and enzymes are made that cannot function properly. Antimetabolites most commonly inhibit the production of purine bases (adenine and guanine in both DNA and RNA) or pyrimidine bases (thymine and cytosine in DNA, and uracil and cytosine in RNA), which are components of the nucleotides that are the building blocks of DNA and RNA; antimetabolites can also replace these nucleotides, making DNA and RNA that work abnormally. Table 3.4 shows subclasses of antimetabolites, gives examples of the drugs, and summarizes their mechanisms of action and their use for treatment of different cancers.

Topoisomerase-Interactive Agents

Topoisomerases are Sites of Chemotherapy Damage. Topoisomerases are enzymes that control the three-dimensional structure of DNA and are necessary for its function. Topoisomerases make cuts in the two strands of DNA that are tightly wound together in a double helix, making breaks that allow the segments of DNA to unwind. After the DNA

Table 3.4 Mechanisms of Action and Diseases treated by Antimetabolites

Subclasses	Mechanisms of Action	Drugs	Diseases Treated
Antifolates	(1) inhibit the dihydrofolate reductase enzyme in folate metabolism and DNA synthesis (2) inhibit purine synthesis	methotrexate (MTX)	acute lymphoblastic leukemia, non-Hodgkin lymphoma, osteosarcoma, head-and-neck, breast, kidney, bladder, and colorectal cancer, choriocarcinoma, autoimmune disease
Fluoropyrimidines	(1) analogues of uracil (2) inhibit the thymidylate synthetase enzyme in DNA synthesis and repair and RNA processing	5-fluorouracil (5-FU)	colorectal and breast cancer, hepatoblastoma
Arabinose nucleosides	(1) analogues of cytosine (2) inhibit the DNA polymerase enzyme in DNA replication and repair	cytarabine (Ara-C)	acute lymphoblastic, acute and chronic myelogenous leukemia, non-Hodgkin lymphoma, multiple myeloma
Deoxycytridines	(1) analogues of cytosine (2) inhibit DNA synthesis and DNA chain lengthening	gemcitabine	pancreas, small bowel, small cell lung, non-small cell lung, and bladder cancer
Thiopurines	(1) analogues of guanine (2) inhibit purine synthesis and metabolism (3) inhibit DNA synthesis	6-mercaptopurine (6-MP)	acute lymphoblastic and myelogenous leukemia

(*Continued*)

Table 3.4 (*Continued*)

Subclasses	Mechanisms of Action	Drugs	Diseases Treated
		6-thioguanine (6-TG)	acute myelogenous leukemia
Fludarabine	(1) analogue of adenosine (2) inhibits the DNA polymerase in DNA synthesis and repair, and DNA chain termination (3) inserts into RNA and inhibits its function (4) interferes with apoptosis	fludarabine	chronic lymphocytic and prolymphocytic leukemia, mantle cell and cutaneous T-cell lymphoma, Waldenström macroglobulinemia
Cladribine	(1) analogue of adenosine (2) inhibits DNA synthesis by terminating DNA chain (3) inhibits the adenosine deaminase enzyme and DNA repair (4) interferes with apoptosis	cladribine (2CdA)	Hairy cell, chronic lymphocytic, and acute myelogenous leukemia, non-Hodgkin lymphoma
2'-deoxycoformycin	(1) analogue of adenosine (2) inhibits DNA synthesis (3) inhibits the adenosine deaminase enzyme and accumulates DNA breaks (4) inhibits RNA synthesis	deoxycoformycin (Pentostatin)	Hairy cell, acute lymphoblastic, chronic lymphocytic, prolymphocytic, and chronic myelogenous leukemia, cutaneous T-cell lymphoma, Langerhans cell histiocytosis

strands have passed through the breaks, the topoisomerases reseal the breaks. There are two types of topoisomerases, type I and type II. The type I enzyme works on single-strand DNA, while the type II enzyme works on double-strand DNA.

Mechanisms of Action. Topoisomerase-interactive agents are plant and fungal products that inhibit the functions of topoisomerases during DNA synthesis. Camptothecins, derived from the *Camptotheca acuminata* plant, prevent the resealing of DNA single-strand breaks made by type I topoisomerase, and stop this enzyme binding to DNA. Podophyllotoxins, derived from mandrake root and May apple, and anthracyclines derived from a *Streptomyces* fungus, inhibit the resealing of DNA cut by type II topoisomerase, and make single-strand and double-strand DNA breaks. Dactinomycin, derived from another *Streptomyces* fungus, inhibits both type I and type II topoisomerase. Table 3.5 shows subclasses of topoisomerase-interactive agents, gives examples of the drugs, and summarizes their mechanisms of action and their use for treatment of different cancers.

Antimicrotubule Agents

Tubulin is a Site of Chemotherapy Damage. Tubulin is a contractile protein, from which microtubules are made. Microtubules are the hollow tubes that form the mitotic spindle, the framework supporting dividing and duplicating chromosomes during mitosis. Microtubules are also necessary for the movements of cells, and the sticking of cells to blood vessels. In addition, microtubules are used to anchor cell membranes and structures, and to perform other transport, secretion, and signal transmission functions.

Table 3.5 Mechanisms of Action and Diseases Treated by Topoisomerase-interactive Agents

Subclasses	Mechanisms of Action	Drugs	Diseases Treated
Podophyllotoxins	(1) inhibit topoisomerase II causing single-strand and double-strand DNA breaks	etoposide (VP-16)	acute lymphoblastic and myelogenous leukemia, Hodgkin and non-Hodgkin lymphoma, neuroblastoma, retinoblastoma, Ewing sarcoma, rhabdomyosarcoma, osteosarcoma, germ cell and brain tumor, small cell lung cancer, Langerhans cell histiocytosis, multiple myeloma, bone marrow transplant
	(2) unwind DNA, interfering with gene transcription and DNA repair	teniposide (VM-26)	
	(3) inhibit DNA synthesis		
Camptothecins	(1) inhibit topoisomerase I, causing single-strand DNA breaks	camptothecin (CPT11) irinotecan	neuroblastoma, retinoblastoma, Ewing sarcoma, rhabdomyosarcoma neuroblastoma, retinoblastoma, Ewing sarcoma, rhabdomyosarcoma, colorectal cancer, brain tumor
	(2) unwind DNA, interfering with gene transcription, DNA replication and repair	topotecan	neuroblastoma, retinoblastoma, Ewing sarcoma, rhabdomyosarcoma, brain tumor
Anthracyclines	(1) bind DNA, preventing its resealing after cut by topoisomerase II	doxorubicin (Adriamycin)	acute lymphoblastic and myelogenous leukemia, Hodgkin and non-Hodgkin lymphoma, neuroblastoma, Ewing sarcoma, osteosarcoma, rhabdomyosarcoma, hepatoblastoma, germ cell
	(2) insert between adjacent		

DNA bases, causing single-strand and double-strand DNA breaks (3) produce reactive free hydroxyl and oxygen radicals, damaging cellular proteins	daunorubicin (Daunomycin) idarubicin	tumor, testicular, breast, ovarian, hepatocellular, and bladder cancer acute lymphoblastic and myelogenous leukemia, non-Hodgkin lymphoma acute lymphoblastic and myelogenous leukemia, non-Hodgkin lymphoma, breast cancer
	epirubicin	acute lymphoblastic and myelogenous leukemias, non-Hodgkin lymphoma, hepatocellular and breast cancer
	dexrazoxane (ICRF187)	prevents reactive free radical damage to the heart from anthracyclines
Anthracenediones — insert between adjacent DNA bases causing single-strand and double-strand DNA breaks	mitoxantrone	acute lymphoblastic and myelogenous leukemia, Hodgkin and non-Hodgkin lymphoma, Ewing sarcoma, neuroblastoma, rhabdomyosarcoma, osteosarcoma, testicular and breast cancer, germ cell tumor
Dactinomycin — (1) inserts between adjacent DNA bases, causing single-strand and double-strand DNA breaks (2) blocks the DNA template used for DNA and RNA synthesis	dactinomycin (Actinomycin D)	Wilms tumor, Ewing sarcoma, osteosarcoma, rhabdomyosarcoma, choriocarcinoma, testicular cancer, germ cell tumor, Kaposi sarcoma

Mechanisms of Action. Antimicrotubule agents are plant products that bind tubulin, interfering with mitotic spindle formation and stopping mitosis when the chromosomes attempt to line up on the mitotic spindle (metaphase). Vinca alkaloids are derived from the periwinkle plant, and taxanes from Pacific yew tree bark. Estramustine, an estradiol hormone combined with a nitrogen mustard, works as an antimicrotubule agent. Table 3.6 shows subclasses of antimicrotubule agents, gives examples of the drugs, and summarizes their mechanisms of action and their use for treatment of different cancers.

Miscellaneous Agents

Mechanisms of Action. These drugs inhibit critical cellular processes. Homoharringtonine is derived from *Cephalotaxus* evergreen trees; bleomycin from another *Streptomyces* fungus; and the asparaginase enzyme from *E. coli* and *Erwinia* bacteria. Synthetic drugs include the antiparasitic drug suramin and the corticosteroids hormones. Table 3.7 shows subclasses of miscellaneous agents, gives examples of the drugs, and summarizes their mechanisms of action and their use for treatment of different cancers.

Principles of Administration of Chemotherapy

Combination Chemotherapy. The use of several drugs together is one of the most important advances in cancer therapy. Several drugs work better than a single drug by attacking different sites or mechanisms, making the combination more effective and less susceptible to drug resistance. The drugs are

Table 3.6 Mechanisms of Action and Diseases Treated by Antimicrotubule Agents

Subclasses	Mechanisms of Action	Drugs	Diseases Treated
Vinca alkaloids	inhibit microtubule function during mitosis	vincristine (VCR)	acute lymphoblastic leukemia, Hodgkin and non-Hodgkin lymphoma, multiple myeloma, neuroblastoma, retinoblastoma, Ewing sarcoma, osteosarcoma, rhabdomyosarcoma, Wilms, germ cell, and brain tumor
		vinblastine (VBL)	Hodgkin lymphoma
		vindesine	acute lymphoblastic leukemia
Taxanes	bind to microtubules, disrupting their function during mitosis	Taxol (paclitaxel)	breast, ovarian, non–small cell lung, small cell lung, and head-and-neck cancer, Kaposi sarcoma
		docetaxel	breast, ovarian, non–small cell lung, small cell lung, and head-and-neck cancer
Estramustines	interfere with the microtubule framework	estramustine phosphate	prostate cancer

Table 3.7 Mechanisms of Action and Diseases Treated by Miscellaneous Anticancer Agents

Subclasses	Mechanisms of Action	Drugs	Diseases Treated
Cephalotaxine esters	produce single-strand and double-strand DNA breaks	homoharringtonine	acute myelogenous and chronic-phase chronic myelogenous leukemia, myelodysplastic syndrome
Suramin	mechanism of action uncertain but binds to many enzymes and plasma proteins	suramin	prostate, adrenal, and renal-cell cancer
Glycopeptide alkaloids	produce single-strand and double-strand DNA breaks	bleomycin	Hodgkin lymphoma, germ cell tumor, osteosarcoma
Hydroxyurea	inhibits the ribonucleotide reductase enzyme essential for DNA synthesis	hydroxyurea (HU)	chronic myelogenous leukemia, malignant melanoma, cervix, head-and-neck, ovarian, and stomach cancer, medulloblastoma
Asparaginase	breaks down and depletes the aminoacid L-asparagine, which	L-asparaginase, long-acting polyethylene	acute lymphoblastic leukemia, non-Hodgkin lymphoma

	normal cells can make but lymphoblasts cannot produce	glycol asparaginase, *Erwinia* asparaginase if allergic to L-asparaginase	
Corticosteroids	mechanism of action uncertain	prednisone, prednisolone, hydrocortisone, dexamethasone (Decadron)	Hodgkin and non-Hodgkin lymphoma, acute lymphoblastic leukemia, brain tumor, Langerhans cell histiocytosis, multiple myeloma
Amifostine	(1) releases free sulfhydryl compounds that destroy tissue-damaging reactive free radicals produced by radiation and chemotherapy (2) donates hydrogen atoms to repair damaged sites (3) binds to toxic breakdown products of drugs	amifostine	prevents anthracycline, platinum, alkylating agent, and radiation damage to kidney, heart, bone marrow, lung, nerves, and bowel

chosen so that they do not have overlapping toxicities. In combination chemotherapy, drugs may be used to block one biochemical step after another (sequential blockade); block two pathways at the same time (concurrent blockade); damage both the biochemical pathway and block its repair mechanism (complementary inhibition); or sensitize cells toward damage by another drug (metabolic sensitization).

Dose Determination. Chemotherapy doses, established by clinical trials, are calculated based on body weight or surface area. Doses are modified for the overweight or underweight. Doses are decreased for reduced kidney, liver, and heart functions or a history of previous increased drug toxicity.

Safe Administration. Drugs may be given by mouth, by intravenous and intramuscular injections, or by lumbar puncture (intrathecal injection). Since many drugs burn skin and tissues if leaked outside the vein, a semipermanent indwelling central venous line (e.g., Portacath™, Broviac™, Hickman™) is often put into the superior vena cava for giving chemotherapy, administering transfusions, antibiotics, hydration, and nutrients, and drawing blood samples. Central lines are kept open with the anticoagulant, heparin, but still has a small risk of blood clots, or infections associated with its use.

Safe Scheduling. Chemotherapy is given in cycles, with two to four weeks of recovery time between treatment cycles to allow the bone marrow and normal cells to recover. Chemotherapy is given only to patients who are reasonably fit, well-nourished, and free of infections, with normal complete blood counts and adequate liver and renal function tests. Chemotherapy that affects the heart, lungs, and hearing are given only if these tests are adequate.

Supportive Therapies. Supportive therapies are important for reducing discomfort and toxicity, to allow patients to tolerate the full course of chemotherapy. Antiemetic drugs are used to prevent nausea and vomiting. Local anesthetics are used to prevent pain from drawing blood samples from veins, accessing central lines, and doing bone marrow and lumbar punctures. Blood and platelet transfusions are used to treat anemia and low platelet counts. Intravenous or tube feeding is used to treat poor nutrition. Antibiotic, antiviral, and antifungal drugs are used to fight bacterial, viral, and fungal infections in patients with low white blood neutrophil counts (neutropenia) and compromised immunity.

Toxicity from Chemotherapy

Chemotherapy Causing Toxicity. Chemotherapy is most toxic for fast-dividing normal cells, such as the skin, hair, mouth, bowel, testes, ovary, lymphatic tissue, and bone marrow precursor cells (stem cells). Fortunately, these normal cells can double their numbers in hours, having an almost unlimited potential to regenerate, and usually recovering from chemotherapy faster than cancer cells. These toxicities are reversible on stopping chemotherapy. Chemotherapy is least toxic for slow- or nondividing normal cells, such as nerve, lung, and kidney cells.

Toxicities Specific to Certain Types of Chemotherapy. Most drugs can cause nausea and vomiting by stimulating the chemoreceptor trigger zone and emesis center in the brain and by slowing the emptying of the stomach and bowels. Vincristine, vinblastine, and platinum compounds can cause constipation by affecting the nerves responsible for bowel activity. When used during pregnancy, alkylating agents and other drugs can cause fetal malformation. Alkylating agents, podophyllotoxins, anthracyclines, and platinum compounds can cause secondary acute myelogenous leukemia in rare instances, and work like radiation to cause mutations and secondary cancers. Anthracyclines and anthracenediones can damage the heart by releasing reactive free radicals that break down heart muscles. Cyclophosphamide and ifosfamide break down into acrolein, which damages the bladder and causes blood in the urine. Bleomycin and alkylating agents such as melphalan, chlorambucil, mitomycin C, carmustine, and busulfan can damage the lungs. Cisplatin and carboplatin can cause hearing loss. Alkylating agents, anthracyclines, and platinum compounds can damage the testes and ovaries, reducing or stopping sperm production in men and stopping menstrual periods and ovulation in women. Hormonal effects often recover quickly after stopping chemotherapy, but sperm production and ovulation may take years to recover or never recover. Prepubertal children are less susceptible to chemotherapy damage to the testes and ovaries. The production of red and white blood cells and platelets from the bone marrow recovers quickly after stopping chemotherapy, but antibody production by B-lymphocytes may take months to recover and cellular immunity mediated by T-lymphocytes may take years to recover.

Classifying Chemotherapy Toxicities by Types, Frequency, and Onset. The types, frequency, and time of onset of the different toxicities for each drug used are now described on treatment consent forms. One way is to use a table to describe the side effects of each drug. The incidence may be expressed as common (21–100 events in 100 treatments), occasional (5–20), or rare (less than 5). The onset may be described as immediate (one or two days after treatment), prompt (within two or three weeks), delayed (later than "immediate" or "prompt"), or late (long after treatment). Table 3.8 shows an example of such a table for etoposide.

Table 3.8 Incidence, Onset, and Types of Side Effects from Etoposide

Onset	Common	Occasional	Rare
Immediate	nausea and vomiting	local ulceration of skin and underlying tissues may occur if medication leaks outside the vein	(1) low blood pressure (2) inability of kidneys to get rid of acid from the body (3) extremely rare life-threatening allergic reaction (4) skin rash
Prompt	decrease in the number of red blood cells, white blood cells, and platelets made in the bone marrow	(1) hair loss which may be prompt or late (2) worsening of the reaction to radiation if radiation given too soon after etoposide (3) diarrhea	(1) damage to nerves that control muscle movements and give awareness of temperature, touch, and pain, or cause tingling and numbness (2) mouth sores
Delayed			
Late			secondary leukemia caused by treatment of a previous cancer or leukemia

Mechanisms of Drug Resistance

Drug resistance describes the processes by which cancers become refractory to chemotherapy, a very important and common problem. Drug resistance can be caused by "upstream" and "downstream" factors that affect how drugs work in cancer cells, as well as mechanisms within cancer cells that allow them to escape the effects of chemotherapy.

Factors "Upstream" to The Cancer Cells. How chemotherapy drugs are delivered and received by the cancer cells depends on tissue factors, tumor factors, drug sanctuaries, and host factors. Tissue factors include the blood and lymphatic supply of the tumor, which delivers drugs to the cancer and are the routes by which cancer cells spread to lymph nodes and other organs. Tumor factors include the ability of the cancer cells to migrate, invade, spread, and implant in other tissues. Drug sanctuaries are due to nature barriers, such as the blood-brain, blood-eye, and blood-testicular barriers, which prevent toxic drugs from entering and damaging sensitive organs like the brain, eye, and testes. Host factors include the patient's ability to activate or inactivate drugs, distribute drugs, break down drugs, and eliminate drugs through the liver and kidneys. All these factors affect whether cancers respond to or fail to respond to chemotherapy.

Factors "Downstream" to The Cancer Cells. Whether or not cancer cells exposed to chemotherapy drugs can eventually be eliminated depends on genetic programs that affect the growth, progression, proliferation, and death of cancer cells. Activation of oncogenes that stimulate cancer growth offsets the tumor-destroying effects of chemotherapy. Inactivation of tumor suppressor genes removes the controls that discourage cancer progression. Activation of cell-proliferation genes encourages the relentless division of cancer cells. Inactivation of proapoptotic genes, which promote cell death, prevents the killing of cancer cells damaged by chemotherapy. Activation of antiapoptotic genes, which prevent cell death, likewise stops the killing of cancer cells that have been damaged by chemotherapy.

Resistance Mechanisms Within Cancer Cells. Resistance mechanisms working within the cancer cells are, by far, the most important factors that allow them to escape damage by chemotherapy. These mechanisms are derived from metabolic pathways that are naturally present in normal cells for protection from damage by natural toxins in the environment. Such drug resistance pathways may become enhanced within cancer cells to block the damaging effects of chemotherapy. Repeated exposure to drugs and radiation can further enhance drug resistance pathways. Some drug resistance pathways are unique to a particular class of drugs. Others, which are most dangerous, can affect many classes of drugs.

Drug Resistance Mechanisms Affecting a Specific Class of Drug. Normal metabolites are carried into cells by transporters. Certain drugs have been designed to use these same transporters, such as methotrexate using the folate transporter, cytarabine using the nucleoside transporter, and Mustargen using the choline transporter. In some cancer cells such transporters become defective and drugs cannot enter, so that the cancer cells are in effect resistant to the chemotherapy. In other cancer cells repair pathways for DNA damage become very active, so that DNA damage caused by alkylating agents and platinum compounds are rapidly repaired, making the cancer cells resistant to these agents.

Drug Resistance Mechanisms Affecting Many Classes of Drugs. Some cancer cells have "drug pumps" within their cell membranes that work like vacuum cleaners to expel many classes of drugs. Since these drug pumps have evolved in normal cells for protection against natural toxins in the environment, the classes of drugs affected by drug pumps are the natural products of plants and fungi. Examples of such drug pumps include P-glycoprotein and the breast cancer resistance protein (BCRP). Other cancer cells may have "drug traps" within their cell membranes, which engulf many classes of natural-product drugs into vacuoles and expel them from the cancer cells. An example of such a drug trap is the multidrug resistance protein (MRP). Still other cancer cells may have "drug carriers" that convey drugs between the cytoplasm and nuclei. An example of such a drug carrier is the lung resistance protein (LRP). Yet other cancer cells may have an increase in the enzymes that alter drug targets, such as the topoisomerase II enzyme, or a decrease of the enzymes that inactivate drugs, such as the glutathione family of enzymes. Table 3.9 summarizes the resistance mechanisms that work within cancer cells both on a specific class of drugs and on many classes of drugs, and gives examples of the drugs affected.

Table 3.9 Mechanisms of Drug Resistance within Cancer Cells

Classes	Mechanisms of Action in Cancer Cells	Targets within Cancer Cells	Specific Drugs or Classes of Drugs Involved in Resistance
Decreased drug concentration within cancer cells	defective transporter for normal metabolites that cannot carry specific drugs into cells	folate transporter nucleoside transporter choline transporter	methotrexate cytarabine mechlorethamine
	"drug pumps" that remove many groups of drugs from within cancer cells	P-glycoprotein "drug pump"	vinca alkaloids, podophyllotoxins, taxanes, anthracyclines, antibiotics, anthracenediones
		breast cancer resistance protein (BCRP) "drug pump"	anthracyclines, camptothecins, anthracenediones
	"drug pumps" that redirect the movements of many groups of drugs within cancer cells	multidrug resistance protein (MRP) "drug trap" that engulfs drugs into vacuoles, and works with the glutathione-S-conjugate transporter to transport drugs out	vinca alkaloids, podophyllotoxins, taxanes, anthracyclines, antibiotics, anthracenediones
		lung resistance protein (LRP) "drug carrier" that controls drug traffic between the nucleus and cytoplasm	anthracyclines, vinca alkaloids
Increased drug break down in	increased inactivation of a specific drug	high inactivating enzyme, bleomycin hydrolase	bleomycin

(Continued)

Table 3.9. (Continued)

Classes	Mechanisms of Action in Cancer Cells	Targets within Cancer Cells	Specific Drugs or Classes of Drugs Involved in Resistance
cancer cells		high inactivating enzyme, aldehyde dehydrogenase	cyclophosphamide
		high inactivating enzyme, cytidine deaminase	cytarabine
Increased repair of drug damage	increased DNA repair for damage caused by specific groups of drugs	increased repair of DNA damaged by drugs in cancer cells	platinum compounds, alkylating agents
Altered sites in cancer cells damaged by drugs	changing activities of cells targeted by a group of drugs	mutation of topoisomerase II drug target	podophyllotoxins, taxanes, anthracyclines, antibiotics, anthracenediones
	increased drug target enzyme for a specific drug	high dihydrofolate reductase enzyme	methotrexate
		high thymidylate synthetase enzyme	5-fluorouracil
		high adenosine deaminase enzyme	2'-deoxycoformycin
Activation of drug resistance genes	amplification of drug resistance genes	increased copies of the P-glycoprotein and MRP genes	vinca alkaloids, podophyllotoxins, taxanes, anthracyclines, antibiotics, anthracenediones
	increased expression of drug resistance genes	increased P-glycoprotein and MRP protein activity	

4. Surgical Oncology

Surgery is the only recourse for cancers that do not respond to chemotherapy or radiation. This localized therapy is successful only if cancers have not spread to other parts of the body and can be removed completely.

Cancer surgery is complete removal of the cancer and adjacent involved lymph nodes and structures in one single piece with no tumors cells at the edges (negative surgical margins). Primary surgery is performed at diagnosis if complete removal of the cancer is thought to be possible. If the cancer is inoperable at diagnosis but shrinks with chemotherapy or radiation, secondary surgery is performed to remove any residual tumor. If the cancer still remains inoperable, alternative chemotherapy or more radiation may be given. Second-look surgery is performed should the cancer respond to the additional treatment. Surgery is important for removing chemotherapy-resistant and radiation-resistant cancer cells, and both dividing cancer cells and nondividing cancer cells that are protected from chemotherapy and radiation.

In children, most cancers are first shrunk with chemotherapy. If the cancer can then be removed completely, the cure rate is better and long-term complications are less. Avoiding radiation is important in children because it stunts growth and produces permanent cosmetic and functional defects. Secondary cancers may also be caused by radiation. Mutilating surgery, however, is not attempted if complete removal is unlikely, since deformities are worse if radiation has to be given on top of extensive surgery.

Table 4.1 Summary of the Timing, Purpose, and Types of Surgery

When	What	How
At diagnosis	confirm diagnosis and test for pathologic, biologic, genetic, and hormonal prognostic markers stage lymph nodes, bone marrow, and cerebrospinal fluid for presence of tumor primary surgery central venous line treat oncological emergencies	(1) closed biopsy that looks for cancer cells in body fluids; or biopsy of the tumor with a needle, with image guidance (ultrasound or CT scan), or through a telescope into the bowel or bladder (endoscopy) (2) open biopsy that removes a piece of tumor (incisional biopsy) or the whole tumor (excisional biopsy) removes operable cancers resistant to chemotherapy and radiation delivery of chemotherapy and supportive therapy (1) severe hemorrhage (2) organ perforation (3) surgery to relieve increased intracranial pressure from brain tumor (ventriculoperitoneal shunt) (4) surgery to relieve spinal cord compression (laminectomy)
After treatment	total removal of cancer, involved lymph nodes, and adjacent structures removal of positive surgical margins second-look surgery after chemotherapy or radiation removal of metastases	aims at achieving negative surgical margins

At relapse	palliative surgery	improves quality of life and relieves pain, obstruction, and severe hemorrhage
At long-term follow-up	reconstructive surgery	(1) corrects postsurgery, postradiation, or postchemotherapy complications (2) restores function (3) corrects defects (4) removes scars
High-risk conditions	prophylactic surgery before genetic cancers develop	(1) removes breasts and ovaries to prevent breast cancer for *BRCA1* or *BRCA2* gene mutations (2) removes ovaries to prevent ovarian cancer in familial ovarian cancer syndrome (3) removes colon with polyps to prevent colon cancer in familial adenomatous polyposis (FAP) syndrome or hereditary nonpolyposis colorectal cancer (HNPCC) (4) removes thyroid gland to prevent medullary thyroid cancer in multiple endocrine neoplasia (MEN) syndrome types 2 and 3
	prophylactic surgery before nongenetic cancers develop	(1) surgical relocation of undescended testes into the scrotum to prevent testicular cancer (2) removes colon to prevent colon cancer in chronic ulcerative colitis with abnormal-looking cells present (dysplasia) (3) removes esophagus to prevent esophageal cancer in chronic inflammation with dysplasia (Barrett esophagus)

Many cancers in adults do not respond to chemotherapy. Radiation is often important for treating these cancers. It is less important to avoid radiation in adults since stunting of growth is not an issue. The bulk of these cancers and involved lymph nodes and adjacent structures are often removed first so as to reduce the tumor volume for radiation. This type of "debulking surgery" may also be performed before bone marrow transplant. Table 4.1 summarizes and gives examples of the types of surgery for cancer.

Surgical Counseling

When informed consent is obtained for surgery, the possible immediate and late complications and rare or unexpected side effects of the procedure, anesthesia, and supportive drugs must be explained. Potential complications of inserted devices, such as clotting or infection in central venous lines, are discussed. Surgeons and anesthetists assess the risk of the procedure and anesthetic risk depending on age, prior medical conditions, and effects of the cancer to decide if local, regional, or general anesthesia should be used.

5. Radiation Therapy

Advances in radiation therapy have greatly improved the cure rates of many cancers, especially those that cannot be removed and do not respond to chemotherapy. Radiation can cure many adults with cervix, larynx, breast, and prostate carcinoma, seminoma, and Hodgkin lymphoma. Radiation can also cure many children with brain tumor, Hodgkin lymphoma, neuroblastoma, rhabdomyosarcoma, Wilms tumor, Ewing sarcoma, and retinoblastoma, but at the price of stunting bone and soft tissue growth and causing permanent cosmetic and functional defects, with learning problems if the brain is radiated. For these reasons, children should be treated with chemotherapy and surgery, and radiation should be avoided if possible. Other long-term effects include cataracts, damage to cornea, dry mouth, blockage of blood vessels of the heart and brain, lung damage, baldness, and sterility. Importantly, radiation may cause up to 5–15 percent secondary cancers in children and adults. To understand how radiation works, it is important to know what radiation is and its effect on cell biology.

Radiation Physics

What is Radiation? There are two types of radiotherapy, electromagnetic and subatomic particles. Electromagnetic radiation is commonly used and consists of x-rays and gamma rays. Subatomic particles are rarely used and consist of electrons, neutrons, negatively charged pi-mesons, heavy-charged α-particles, atomic nuclei, and protons. The energy from radiation is called photons. As photon energy passes through tissues, electrons rotating around the atomic nuclei are ejected, creating more photon energy that further ejects more electrons. The photon energy produced on absorption of radiation is measured in centiGrays (cGys), previously called rads. X-rays are produced by machines, which before 1960 were low-energy or orthovoltage (100–400 thousand electron volts), but nowadays are high-energy or supravoltage (2–25 million electron volts). Gamma rays are produced when the nucleus of a radioisotope, such as ^{60}cobalt, breaks up. Radiation energy gets less as it penetrates tissues, so superficial tissues receive more radiation than deeper tissues. Different types of radiation also penetrate tissues differently. Low-energy radiation causes severe skin damage and is absorbed by bone more than soft tissue, whereas high-energy radiation spares the skin and is absorbed by bone and soft tissue equally.

Radiation Biology

Cell Injury.   On absorption of radiation, water molecules within cells eject electrons to produce ions, a process called ionization. This is why radiation is sometimes called ionizing radiation. Ions break down into a free hydroxyl radical, which is highly reactive and can cause tissue damage. Reactive free radicals also break chemical bonds and damage DNA. Some DNA injuries can be repaired but others cannot, causing errors during DNA synthesis at cell division and resulting in cell death. Cells damaged by radiation break up, die, age rapidly, or lose their ability to divide. Some cells die rapidly, but others die when they next divide, divide abnormally, fail to divide, or produce daughter cells that cannot divide.

Cell Death.   Below certain radiation doses cell injury is not lethal because repair is possible, but above these levels radiation is lethal and cell death inevitable. Both normal cells and cancer cells go through the cell cycle, the different phases a cell goes through during its lifetime. Cells are most sensitive during mitosis (M phase), early DNA synthesis (early S phase), and during protein and RNA synthesis just before mitosis (G_2 phase), but most resistant during late DNA synthesis (late S phase) and during protein and RNA synthesis in late G_1 before DNA synthesis. Cells in the G_0 phase are resting and not dividing, so they cannot be killed by radiation. Some cancers divide so rapidly that they appear not to respond to radiation, because cell division is faster than cell kill.

Cell Repair.   Different types of normal tissues and different cancers respond differently to radiation. This is known as susceptibility to radiation damage. The total dose of radiation depends on the susceptibility of the cancer, as well as the susceptibility of adjacent normal tissues. The higher the radiation dose, the greater is the damage to both cancer cells and normal cells, and the less likely is their repair and recovery. The effectiveness and toxicity also depend on how the radiation is given, that is, over a number of days (fractionation), and the total duration of radiation. Fractionation is a way to protect normal tissues from radiation trauma by allowing cells to divide and move in to repopulate the damaged area.

Radiosensitivity.   Cancers are called sensitive if they respond to radiation doses that are tolerated. At these radiation doses, more cancer cells than normal cells should be damaged and killed, and cancer cell repair and recovery should not be faster than cancer cell killing.

Radioresistance.   Cancers are called resistant if they respond only to higher radiation doses that are poorly tolerated; if more normal cells than cancer cells are damaged and killed; or if cancer cell repair and recovery are faster than cancer cell killing.

Importance of Oxygen. Radiation is three times more effective with oxygen present than without. This means that in a low oxygen environment, the radiation dose must be three times higher to kill as many cancer cells. This is because oxygen protects the reactive free radicals released by radiation that damage the DNA of cancer cells. In practice, low oxygen in anemic patients undergoing radiation is prevented by blood transfusions that increase the oxygen carried by the red blood cells. However, extra oxygen at higher pressure (hyperbaric oxygen) has not been shown to make radiation more effective. Another possibility is to use drugs called radiosensitizers to make cancer cells more sensitive to radiation.

Radiosensitizers. Radiosensitizers mimic the effect of oxygen in increasing radiation damage. The most common radiosensitizer is the nitroimidazole compound misonidazole. However, some radiosensitizers are themselves toxic and can damage normal cells, so no net benefit may result. Other radiosensitizers insert themselves onto the DNA of cancer cells, resulting in increased DNA damage by radiation and decreased DNA repair. These radiosensitizers include bromodeoxyuridine, iododeoxyuridine, and compounds that are structurally similar to thymidine (analogues) so that they could inhibit its normal functions.

Radioprotectors. Radioprotectors are drugs that protect normal cells (more than cancer cells) from damage by reactive free radicals released by radiation. Glutathione is a natural radioprotector produced by the body. The cysteamine analogue, Amifostine, is an experimental radioprotector. Amifostine is a prodrug, which means that it must first be activated in the body before it works. The alkaline phosphatase enzyme activates Amifostine, which releases sulfhydryl compounds that can destroy the reactive free radicals produced by radiation. Amifostine also protects against reactive free radicals released by chemotherapy, such as anthracyclines, platinums, and alkylating agents.

Other Effects of Radiation. Radiation has other adverse effects. It stimulates oncogenes, genes that promote cancer. Increased oncogene activity disrupts the signaling pathways that coordinate the functions of body cells. Radiation increases the production of tumor necrosis factor-α, a growth factor that causes cell damage; stimulates protein synthesis and inhibits protein breakdown; and damages blood vessels, releasing angiogenic factors that make more new blood vessels.

Principles of Radiation Therapy

Safe Administration. When informed consent is obtained for radiation, the possible immediate and late complications are explained. Safe administration of radiation requires careful planning and meticulous administration.

Radiation Planning. Planning determines the total dose, area radiated (field), the cancer and adjacent involved tissues with a margin of normal tissues (volume), daily fractions, and duration of radiation. Simulation with CT scan determines all the positions of radiation beams to the radiated volume when the patient is placed in the treatment position. The radiation physicist draws a computer map of the exact amounts of radiation given to the cancer and the surrounding normal tissues. Laser lights are used to define the converging and diverging radiation beams on the patient's skin, which is then tattooed. A custom-made plaster cast is fitted so that positioning is reproducible for every day of radiation. Custom-made blocks attached to a tray are fitted onto the beam source of the radiation machine, so that shielding of normal tissues is reproducible daily.

Radiation Administration.   Radiation must be given with the patient keeping absolutely still. Parents talk to older children on an intercom system to keep them still during treatment, but young children have to be sedated or put under general anesthesia. X-ray films are taken with the patient in position on the first day of treatment and then periodically, to check against the planning and simulation images. If there is a problem with the patient setup, the radiation oncologist observes the treatment and discusses the solution with the patient or parents.

Dose Determination.   The radiation schedule is the total dose, number of fractions, and treatment duration. Radiation schedules have been determined for different types of cancers, and are designed to give the best local tumor control with the lowest immediate and late complications in normal tissues. Radiation is usually given as a single daily fraction of 150–200 cGys over a few minutes, five days a week for five to eight weeks, to a total dose of 4,000–7,000 cGys, depending on different cancer types.

Radiation Fractionation.   Greater fractionation allows time for normal tissues to repair, by cells dividing and moving in to repopulate the damaged area. However, sparing normal tissues also means more recovery of cancer cells, so that higher total doses and longer treatments are needed for cancer control. Greater fractionation does have certain benefits. More oxygen goes into low-oxygen areas, making radiation more effective at killing well-oxygenated cancer cells. Cancer cells have time to go back to cell cycle phases where they are more sensitive to radiation. An unconventional way to give radiation is called hyperfractionation, which means that more than one fraction is given daily. It is a way to give higher total doses, which is tolerated by normal tissues, without prolonging treatment. In practice, twice-daily 75–100 cGy-fractions are used during hyperfractionation instead of conventional once-daily 150–200 cGy-fractions, allowing repair of normal cells but not of cancer cells. Hyperfractionation is experimental, and benefit has to be confirmed to justify this more costly and time-consuming procedure. Hypofractionation means using fewer but larger fractions, generally during palliative radiation. Split-course radiation means a break in the middle of treatment, generally for major toxicity in patients.

Chemotherapy Given with Radiation. This has several advantages. Cure rates are higher without increased toxicity. Hard-to-treat cancers such as breast, colon, and head-and-neck cancers respond better. However, some drugs, such as doxorubicin, daunorubicin, and dactinomycin, can sensitize normal cells to radiation in what is known as the radiation-recall phenomenon. There is an acute reaction with skin and muscle breakdown, and radiation damage to lung, kidney, liver, and bowel.

Surgery Combined with Radiation. This has several advantages. Less extensive surgery is needed, without sacrificing surrounding vital organs. Removing the bulk of the cancer makes radiation work better. The oxygen supply within smaller tumor volumes is better, making radiation more effective. Radiation may be preoperative, rendering inoperable cancers operable, and sterilizing tumor edges to reduce tumor spread during surgery. Preoperative radiation, however, may confuse surgical staging, and possibly delay surgery. Postoperative radiation, for patients with incomplete tumor removal, treats smaller volumes and allows wounds to be fully healed before radiation. Postoperative radiation, however, changes blood and oxygen supply to cancer cells and cannot protect against tumor spread during surgery; also, scar tissues may tether down the bowel to cause more radiation damage.

Palliative Radiation.   Once given, radiation cannot be repeated without drastic complications. Radiated tissues "remember" the previous insult. Repeat radiation results in irreparable tissue breakdown and blood vessel blockage, causing brain damage, death from damage to brainstem cardiovascular and respiratory centers, paralysis from spinal cord damage, severe damage to the eye, heart, lung, kidney, liver, bowel, ovary, and testes, limb contracture, and pain from blood vessel and nerve damage. Since these complications usually occur after years, palliative radiation for short-term control of pain and symptoms is acceptable in patients with relapsed and progressing cancers.

Radiation Techniques

Teletherapy and Brachytherapy.   Teletherapy is external-beam radiation, using a machine that sends out x-rays, gamma rays, or electron beams, radiating the tumor volume and adjacent normal tissues. Brachytherapy is putting a radioactive device on or inside the tumor volume, so that adjacent normal tissues receive little radiation.

Toxicity from Radiation Therapy

Genetic Predisposition to Radiation-Induced Cancers.   Some mutations increase the risk of radiation-induced cancers. These mutations involve tumor suppressor genes whose main function is to prevent cancer. One mutation on one chromosome does not cause cancer, but a double mutation of the

Table 5.1 Types of Radiation, Mechanisms of Action, and Advantages and Disadvantages

Classes	Mechanism of Action	Types	Advantages and Disadvantages
Teletherapy	external-beam radiation from a machine	pre-1960 orthovoltage machines (100–400 KEV energy range) produce X-rays	supravoltage is better than orthovoltage, causing less skin damage and lower doses to bone; penetrates deeply into tissues; radiation beams are well defined, allowing daily treatments to be more accurate and reproducible with shorter daily fraction times
		[60]cobalt radioisotope supravoltage machines (1.25 MeV energy range) produce gamma rays	
		linear accelerator supravoltage machines (2–25 MeV photon energy range) produce X-rays	
		linear accelerator supravoltage machines (10–25 MeV range) produce electron beam radiation	advantages include concentration of radiation just below the skin with little penetration into tissues; disadvantages include greater skin damage and absorption into bone, and poorly defined radiation beams
		high-energy cyclotron machines produce proton beam radiation	experimental radiation that does not depend on oxygen to be effective, and can be used for stereotactic radiation to give high doses localized to small tumors with no radiation scattered to adjacent normal tissues

(Continued)

Table 5.1 (*Continued*)

Classes	Mechanism of Action	Types	Advantages and Disadvantages
		cyclotron machines (7–14 MeV energy range) produce neutron beam radiation	experimental radiation that does not depend on oxygen to be effective, and penetrates only shallowly
		linear accelerator supravoltage machines or proton and gamma knife machines delivering narrow beams from all directions to focus on the tumor volume and avoid adjacent healthy tissues (stereotactic radiation)	high-dose radiation, best for treating cancers smaller than 5 cm, that avoids radiating normal tissues
		linear accelerator supravoltage machines using many radiation fields each with a different intensity profile determined by a computer program (intensity-modulated radiation therapy, or IMRT)	high-dose radiation, best for treating cancers smaller than 6 cm, that avoids radiating normal tissues
Brachytherapy	radioactive device placed on or	^{192}iridium or ^{125}iodine radioactive implants placed inside tumors or	high-dose radiation for cancers smaller than 5–10 cm in the bladder, uterus, cervix, and

inside the tumor volume or radioisotope taken internally	within a body cavity	vagina, with little damage to adjacent normal tissues
	^{60}cobalt, ^{125}iodine, ^{192}iridium or ^{109}ruthenium radioisotope put in a mold that is placed on the tumor surface	high-dose radiation for cancers smaller than 1.6 cm, with little radiation scattered to normal tissues because the radioisotope is placed in a gold-shielded mold
	^{131}iodine radioisotope given intravenously or taken orally	thyroid gland first removed to cause hypothyroidism, so that the remaining thyroid tissues and metastases take up ^{131}iodine avidly

Table 5.2 Acute and Chronic Damage to Normal Tissues, Prevention and Support

Tissues	Acute Damage	Chronic Damage	Prevention and Support
Skin	redness, dryness, flaking, increased skin pigments, and ulcers, starting in days to weeks	decreased skin pigments, thinning of skin, dilated blood vessels, and scarring	avoid sunlight and medications that sensitize the skin, causing radiation-recall phenomenon due to dactinomycin, doxorubicin, daunorubicin; clean skin with dilute hydrogen peroxide, apply nothing on the skin until after radiation, when steroid and lanolin may be applied
Hair	hair loss, starting in weeks	permanent hair loss	none
Mouth, esophagus, stomach, and bowel	redness, ulcers, nausea and vomiting, loss of appetite, regurgitation of stomach acid, yeast infection, small and large bowel inflammation, and diarrhea, starting in days to weeks	small bowel obstruction from scar tissues tethering down the bowels	avoid radiosensitizing drugs such as fluorouracil, methotrexate, doxorubicin, daunorubicin, and dactinomycin around radiation; use dilute hydrogen peroxide mouthwash, oral or local painkillers, liquid antacids, nausea medicine, and treat yeast infection; provide intravenous or tube feeding if cannot eat or drink
Salivary and tear glands	dry eye and mouth, starting in days to weeks	permanent dry eye and mouth	shield salivary and lacrimal glands if possible during radiation

Thyroid gland	rare inflammation of thyroid gland, starting in weeks	low thyroid hormone, and benign or malignant thyroid tumors	shield thyroid gland if possible during radiation
Other endocrine glands	early complications are rare	shortness from low growth hormone, poor thyroid hormone production from low thyroid-stimulating hormone, adrenal failure from low adrenocorticotrophic hormone, poor progesterone and estrogen production from low follicle-stimulating hormone and luteinizing hormone, and precocious puberty from high prolactin	shield pituitary gland and the hypothalamus if possible during brain radiation
Bone marrow	low lymphocyte, neutrophil, red blood, and platelet counts, starting in days to weeks	red blood, neutrophil, and platelet counts recover in 1 month, B-lymphocytes in 1–3 months, but T-lymphocytes take 1–5 years to recover	blood and platelet transfusions for anemia and low platelet counts, intravenous antibiotics for fever and neutropenia or infections, and gamma globulin to prevent severe or fatal viral infection from low antibody production by B cells

(Continued)

Table 5.2 (*Continued*)

Tissues	Acute Damage	Chronic Damage	Prevention and Support
Eye	dry eye and corneal ulcers, starting in weeks	retina damage, cataract formation, chronic corneal ulcers	keep eye open during radiation, and treat corneal ulcers to prevent permanent corneal damage
Ear	none	damage to the hearing and balancing functions of the inner ear	keep total doses of hearing-damaging cisplatin and carboplatin low, and avoid other drugs that damage hearing, including some antibiotics
Lung	cough, shortness of breath, and fever from inflammation of the lungs, starting in weeks to months	scarring so that lungs cannot stretch properly; oxygen and carbon dioxide diffuse through the lungs poorly	avoid radiosensitizing drugs such as bleomycin, doxorubicin, daunorubicin, and dactinomycin around radiation; keep total bleomycin doses low; treat lung inflammation with steroids; never ever smoke
Heart	chest pain, fever, and shortness of breath from acute inflammation of the pericardium, starting in weeks to months	scarring of the pericardium and heart muscles, narrowing of coronary blood vessels with increased risk of heart attacks	avoid radiosensitizing drugs such as doxorubicin, daunorubicin, and dactinomycin around radiation; keep total doxorubicin and daunorubicin doses low; never ever smoke
Liver	inflammation of the liver, and blockage of small	veno-occlusive disease, scarring and cirrhosis of the	avoid radiosensitizing drugs such as methotrexate, doxorubicin, daunorubicin,

	blood vessels in the liver (veno-occlusive disease), causing abnormal liver function tests, low platelet count, and free fluid in the abdomen, starting in weeks to months	liver and liver failure	and dactinomycin around radiation; avoid viral infections that damage the liver, such as cytomegalic inclusion virus disease, infectious mononucleosis caused by the Epstein-Barr virus, and hepatitis A, B, and C infections
Kidney	swelling, fluid retention, protein in urine, hypertension, and abnormal kidney function tests from inflammation of kidney, starting in weeks to months	abnormal kidney function tests, kidney failure, hypertension, and breaking up of red blood cells in hemolytic anemia from scarring of renal tubules and blockage of the blood vessels of the kidney (veno-occlusive disease)	avoid radiosensitizing drugs such as doxorubicin, daunorubicin, and dactinomycin around radiation; keep total doses low for kidney-damaging cisplatin and carboplatin, and some antibiotics and antifungal drugs; never ever smoke; do not neglect treating hypertension and diabetes mellitus
Brain	fever, sleepiness, tiredness, and poor appetite from reduced blood flow and damage of brain tissues (postradiation syndrome), starting in weeks to months	brain tissue breakdown, memory loss, intellectual deficit, learning problems in children, and gray and white matter damage (leucoencephalopathy) from brain radiation combined	avoid methotrexate especially in higher doses around radiation; steroid therapy for postradiation syndrome and damaged brain tissues; surgical removal of damaged area of brain tissues

(Continued)

Table 5.2 (*Continued*)

Tissues	Acute Damage	Chronic Damage	Prevention and Support
		with methotrexate, causing seizures, neurological problems, and narrowing of blood vessels with increased risk of strokes	
Spinal cord	reduced blood flow and damage of spinal cord tissues (Lhermitte syndrome) causing sharp shock-like pain in the limbs on bending the neck, starting in weeks to months	damage of the spinal cord, paralysis, and nerve damage pain (Brown-Séquard syndrome)	steroid therapy for postradiation damaged spinal cord tissues
Ovary	stopping of menstrual periods, starting in month	never going into puberty, menstrual periods stop, early menopause, low estrogen and progesterone production by the ovary, no ovulation, and sterility	surgically relocate or shield one or both ovaries from radiation if possible; freeze-preserve a piece of ovary before chemotherapy and radiation

Testes	low sperm production, starting in weeks to month	low testosterone production by the testes, no sperm produced, low sperm counts or abnormal-looking sperm produced, and sterility	shield one or both testes from radiation if possible; freeze-preserve sperm before chemotherapy and radiation
Limbs and skeleton	none	growing soft tissues and bones of children stop growing, curvature of the spine, cosmetic defects of the face and body, limb shortening and contractures, joint problems, nerve damage pain	use only chemotherapy and surgery to treat cancer and avoid radiation in growing children if possible
Cancer and leukemia induction	none	skin, airway, bowel, thyroid gland, salivary gland, and breast cancers, glioblastoma multiforme and malignant astrocytoma of brain, and bone and soft tissue sarcoma	since radiation causes 5–15% long-term risk for developing secondary cancers and leukemia, certain chemotherapy that adds to this risk should be avoided if possible, such as alkylating agents, anthracyclines, podophyllotoxins, and platinum compounds

same gene on the other chromosome will cause the loss of tumor suppressor activity and allow cancer to develop. The inheritable form of retinoblastoma is due to a double mutation of the *RB1* gene. Every cell in the bodies of these patients already carries one copy of the *RB1* gene mutation. A second mutation in the same region will cause bone and soft tissue sarcoma, skin cancer, or brain tumors, particularly after radiation or alkylating agent chemotherapy that causes a lot of mutations. A *p53* gene mutation is the cause of the Li-Fraumeni syndrome, which predisposes to radiation-induced sarcoma and other cancers. A *PTCH* gene mutation in patients with the basal cell nevus carcinoma syndrome causes increased susceptibility to radiation, with development of skin cancer and the brain tumor medulloblastoma. An *ATM* gene mutation in patients with ataxia telangietasia predisposes them to developing leukemia and lymphoma. Ataxia telangietasia, Blooms syndrome, Fanconi syndrome, and xeroderma pigmentosum are syndromes with fragile chromosomes, causing defective DNA repair and increased susceptibility to leukemia and cancer due to radiation and alkylating agent chemotherapy.

Acute and Chronic Toxicity from Radiation.   Different tissues tolerate radiation differently. In general, nerve tissues, bone, bowel, eye, heart, blood vessels, muscles, and connective tissues tolerate more radiation than skin, lung, kidney, bone marrow, ovary, testes, and endocrine glands. Prophylactic therapy may reduce suffering and prevent severe and permanent complications.

6. Biologic and Other Therapies

Biologic therapy is treating cancer by manipulating immune responses, or using mammalian products for therapy. Biologic therapy includes immunotherapy and hormonal therapy. Related fields discussed in this Chapter include bone marrow transplant, supportive therapy, alternative therapy, and palliative therapy.

Principles of Biologic Therapy

Biologic therapy works on both the cancer and cells that have spread throughout the body, and is effective against both dividing and nondividing cancer cells. However, most biological therapies are still experimental and cannot replace surgery, chemotherapy, and radiation. They are useless when the tumor load is large at diagnosis and relapse. They work best when surgery, chemotherapy, and radiation have destroyed the bulk of tumor and there is only minimal disease remaining.

Immunotherapy

Biology of Immunotherapy. The function of the immune system is to eliminate what it recognizes as nonself but to tolerate self. Cancer cells are altered by mutations so that they contain molecules with specific characteristics (antigens) considered nonself by the immune system. The killing of cancer cells involves both the cellular and humoral components of the immune system. The cellular components consist of lymphocytes, monocytes, macrophages, and cells with long cytoplasmic processes for capturing and presenting antigens (dendritic cells), which are involved in both recognizing and killing tumor cells. The humoral components include cytokines, interferons (IFNs), and interleukins (ILs), natural hormonelike immune substances produced by the body that are involved in the killing process. The killing of cancer cells is a complex process. First, cancer cells have to be recognized by their nonself antigens. Then the killing mechanisms must be switched on. Finally, killed cancer cells have to be disposed of. Tumor cells can sometimes escape recognition and destruction by the immune system, allowing the cancer to grow and progress. Immunotherapy acts by making the cancer cells look even more nonself, enhancing their recognition by the cellular immune system. Immunotherapy also acts by boosting the cellular immune killing system to destroy the cancer cells.

Cellular Immune Recognition System. Lymphocytes are involved in killing cancer cells, which they must first recognize as nonself. Lymphocytes consist of T cells and B cells that are identifiable by their markers, and null cells that have no such markers. These markers, called clusters of differentiation or CD, distinguish lymphocytes that have different functions, such as CD8 killer T cells, CD4 helper T cells, CD4/CD8 suppressor T cells, CD19/CD20 antibody-producing B cells, and null natural killer cells (NK cells). The antigens specific to cancer cells are recognizable by T-cell receptors or antibodies. These tumor antigens are recognized and captured by structures called antigen-binding sites. Other cells involved in recognizing tumor cells are the antigen-presenting cells (APCs), which include monocytes, macrophages, dendritic cells, and switched-on B cells and T cells. Special molecules, called major histocompatibility complexes (MHC), also help the immune system recognize tumor cells in one of two ways. In the direct way, Class I MHC molecules on the tumor cells present their antigens as small chains of amino acids, called recognition peptides, which are recognized by the T-cell receptors on CD8 T cells. In the indirect way, Class II MHC molecules on the APCs capture recognition peptides, presenting them for recognition by the T-cell receptors on CD4 T cells.

Cellular Immune Killing System.   During the process of recognizing tumor antigens, T cells become switched on or activated. Activated CD8 T cells release granules that dissolve tumor cells or trigger death receptors on the tumor cells to turn on the apoptosis process (see chapter 9). Activated CD4 T cells can directly kill tumor cells. Other killing processes are also activated, such as B-cell production of antibodies, macrophage ingestion of tumor cells, and release of cytokines. The activated T cells in turn stimulate the release, multiplication, and maturation of other T cells. There are also various ligand signals on antigen-presenting cells that can react with different receptors on the T cell to switch on naïve T cells not previously exposed to tumor antigens.

Roles of Cytokines.   Cytokines are natural hormonelike immune substances produced by white blood cells. They include interferons (IFNs), interleukins (ILs), tumor necrosis factor (TNF), and colony-stimulating factors (CSFs). IFNs, ILs, and TNF are important for killing tumor cells and for regulating the activities of lymphocytes and antigen-presenting cells that recognize and kill tumor cells. Colony-stimulating factors stimulate the recovery of bone marrow cells: G-CSF for neutrophils, GM-CSF for neutrophils, monocytes, erythrocytes, and megakaryocytes, and M-CSF for monocytes and macrophages.

Interferons in the Humoral Immune Killing System.
Interferons (IFN-α, IFN-β and IFN-γ) are natural proteins
essential for life. They have many functions, including switching on DNA transcription to make mRNA and controlling
the signal pathways used by cells. Interferons are also involved
in killing tumor cells by acting on cell division, differentiation, and apoptosis. They also help recognize tumor antigens
by switching on important immune-related molecules, such as
Class I or Class II MHCs, T-cell receptors, and molecules
inside tumor cells (intracellular adhesion molecules, or
ICAMs). They help kill tumor cells by mobilizing other
immune killer cells such as macrophages, monocytes, dendritic cells, T cells, B cells and NK cells. Interferons can also
turn off angiogenesis and destroy tumor blood vessels.

Anticancer Opportunities of Interferons.   IFN-α has been
produced artificially and is presently used in clinical trials for
Kaposi sarcoma, carcinoid, melanoma, bladder and renal cell
carcinoma, non-Hodgkin lymphoma, and hairy cell and chronic
myelogenous leukemia. IFN-α is used with a vitamin A
derivative (retinoic acid) for cervix, renal cell, and airway
and gastrointestinal carcinoma. IFN-α is also used with
chemotherapy, interleukin-2, the antiestrogen tamoxifen,
or steroids, for malignant melanoma and non-Hodgkin
lymphoma. IFN-γ has been synthesized and is presently
used in clinical trials for renal cell carcinoma, and with
chemotherapy or vaccines for neuroblastoma and malignant
melanoma.

Interleukins in the Humoral Immune Killing System.   Interleukins are so called because they work in between leukocytes.
IL-2 is most important member of this family of natural
growth factors. IL-2 is involved in recognizing and killing
tumor cells. The IL-2 receptor can be switched on by signals
from the T-cell receptor; IL-2 in turn signals T cells and NK

cells to recognize tumor antigens and kill tumor cells. IL-2 acts as a growth factor to keep T cells dividing. IL-2 also releases tumor necrosis factor, other interleukins, lymphotoxin, and nitrous oxide that help kill tumor cells.

Anticancer Opportunities of Interleukins. Cells with antitumor activity may be used to treat patients with cancer in a process called adoptive immunotherapy. These cells are made more potent if used together with cytokines. For example, synthesized IL-2 is presently used with cultured lymphokine-activated killer lymphocytes (LAK cells) in clinical trials for non-Hodgkin and Hodgkin lymphoma, melanoma, and renal cell, non–small cell lung, colorectal, and ovarian carcinoma. IL-2 is also used with cultured tumor-infiltrating lymphocytes (TILs), monoclonal antibodies, and vaccines or chemotherapy for metastatic melanoma and renal cell carcinoma.

Antibodies in the Humoral Immune Killing System. Immunoglobulins are antibodies produced by B cells. Immunoglobulins are made up of a κ or λ light chain and a heavy chain, each with a variable region containing two antigen-binding sites and a constant region. The constant region differs in each of the five classes of immunoglobulins: early-onset IgM antibodies; late-onset IgG antibodies; IgA antibodies in saliva, breast milk, and bowel secretions; IgE antibodies in allergic reactions; and IgD antibodies with unknown functions. The most important immunoglobulins that help recognize and kill tumor cells, IgM and IgG, can be found on the surfaces of B cells. These immunoglobulin molecules have antigen-binding sites that bind to specific recognition regions on tumor cells. They then trigger NK cells and macrophages to kill the tumor cells, and help macrophages to ingest and dispose of them. They also switch on complement, a substance that promotes reactions between antigens and antibodies. Monoclonal antibodies may be used to treat patients with cancer in a process called passive immunotherapy. Antibodies are called monoclonal if they are synthesized by hybridomas, which are artificial tumors made by fusing plasma cell tumors with antibody-producing B cells. Parts of antibodies are also useful for cancer treatment, such as the carboxyl end of heavy chains (called Fc fragments), amino ends of heavy chains (Fab fragments), and the Fab fragment linked to part of the Fc fragment, called $F(ab')_2$ fragments.

Anticancer Opportunities of Monoclonal Antibodies. Monoclonal antibodies are presently used in many clinical trials to kill tumor cells.

- Antibody-dependent cellular cytotoxicity reaction: the Fab region of the antibody is bound to a tumor antigen at the same time that its Fc region is bound to a tumor Fc receptor. Examples of such antibodies are anti-CD20 (rituximab) for CD20-positive B-cell lymphoma, leukemia, and multiple myeloma; anti-HER2/neu (trastuzumab) for HER2/neu-positive breast carcinoma; and anti-GD2 or anti-GD3 for GD2-positive neuroblastoma or GD3-positive melanoma.
- Bispecific antibody: an antibody that reacts with both a tumor antigen and a killer cell trigger molecule. An example of such an antibody is 2B1, which reacts with the HER2/neu breast cancer antigen and with Fc receptors of killer cells.
- Immunocytokine therapy: an antibody fused with IL-2 that stimulates an inflammatory response, attracting inflammatory cells to migrate in and kill tumor cells.
- Antigrowth factor receptor antibody therapy: antibody that stops growth factor receptor-binding, inhibiting the cancer-stimulating ability of the growth factor. An example of such an antibody is MAB225, which prevents epidermal

growth factor from binding to receptors in breast, prostate, head-and-neck, and non–small cell lung carcinoma.

• Anti-idiotype antibody therapy: the idiotype is the antigen-binding site of an antibody called, for example, Ab#1. When Ab#1 binds to a tumor antigen, it induces an anti-idiotype antibody, Ab#2. Ab#2 can be used to immunize patients with cancer, producing an anti-anti-idiotype antibody, Ab#3. Ab#3 in turn can bind to the original tumor antigen, setting off a series of immune reactions that kill tumor cells. An example of such an antibody is anti-CD52 (Campath-1) for CD52-positive melanoma, colorectal carcinoma, and B-cell lymphoma and leukemia.

• Radioimmunoconjugate therapy: a radioisotope attached to an antibody that radiates the tumor cells. An example of such an antibody is ^{131}iodine/anti-CD20 for CD20 B-cell lymphoma and leukemia.

• Immunotoxin therapy: a toxin attached to an antibody that poisons the tumor cells. An example of such an antibody is ricin A-chain/anti-CD22 for CD22 B-cell lymphoma.

• Chemoconjugate therapy: a chemotherapy drug attached to an antibody that destroys the tumor cells. An example of such an antibody is doxorubicin/BR96 for refractory leukemia and cancer.

Cancer Vaccines used to Induce Immune Killing.
Immunization with vaccines has long been used to treat patients with cancer in a process called active immunotherapy. Initially, bacteria such as bacillus Calmette-Guérin or *Corynebacterium parvum*, or chemicals such as levamisole, are used to induce a nonspecific T-cell response against the cancer. Nowadays, vaccines are used to immunize patients against their

own cancers. These vaccines are made from cancer cells that are altered by chemicals, radiation, or mutations, and made more reactive by the insertion of proteins, DNA, RNA, viruses, or bacteria. Vaccine activity is further enhanced with chemicals such as Freund's adjuvant, cytokines such as IL-2 or IL-12, or dendritic cells. These vaccines induce a more potent anticancer immune reaction, producing more CD8 and CD4 T cells that recognize and kill tumor cells, and activating CD4 T cells to secrete more IFN-γ and IL-2 that help the killing process.

Anticancer Opportunities of Cancer Vaccines.   Cancer vaccines are presently used in clinical trials for melanoma, follicular lymphoma, and prostate, cervix, non–small cell lung, renal cell, and colon carcinoma. Cancer vaccines may potentially prevent cancers induced by infectious agents, such as stomach cancer from the *Helicobacter pylori* bacteria, cervix cancer from papillomavirus, liver cancer from hepatitis B and C, Kaposi sarcoma and non-Hodgkin lymphoma from human immunodeficiency virus (HIV) and herpes type 8, adult T-cell leukemia from human T-cell lymphotrophic virus I, and lymphoma from Epstein-Barr virus infection. At present, there are only clinical trials for hepatitis B and papillomavirus infections.

Hormonal Therapy

Biology of Hormonal Therapy.   Hormones stimulate the growth of the hormone-sensitive tissues of the breast, uterus, and prostate gland. Cancers that arise in these organs may still be hormone-dependent: their growth and spread are stimulated by hormones. Hormone-dependent cancers have receptors that recognize specific hormones.

Hormone Receptors. Many hormone receptors are tyrosine kinase enzymes. A hormone receptor is a protein that spans the cell membrane, with a pair of ligand-binding sites outside the cell and a pair of tyrosine kinase sites inside the cell. Their main function is to transmit signals from outside the cell to inside the cell. When hormones react with their receptors, many important pathways inside the cells become switched on.

Estrogen and Progesterone. The ovary makes estrogen and progesterone before menopause, but after menopause the adrenal gland makes estrogen and progesterone from androgens by the aromatization process. Estrogen and progesterone regulate the growth, differentiation, and survival of breast and uterine tissues that have estrogen receptors (ER) and progesterone receptors (PR). About two-thirds of breast and uterine carcinoma also have such receptors, and remain dependent on estrogen and progesterone. ER-positive and PR-positive breast carcinoma have a better prognosis because they respond to hormone manipulation therapy. Hormone receptors are regulated by many signals, such as signals from genes (e.g., cyclin) and growth factors (e.g., epidermal growth factor) that control cell cycle activities. In particular, the epidermal growth factor receptor family is important in breast carcinoma because one family member, HER2/neu, is associated with hormone independence and poor prognosis. However, an antibody called trastuzumab (Herceptin) has been developed against HER2/neu that is able to block HER2/neu activity and prevent progression of breast carcinoma. Hormone manipulation to treat breast and uterine carcinoma includes removing organs that secrete hormones or using antihormones to block hormone production or change the way hormones work.

Estrogen-blocking Therapy. Estrogen-blockage therapy is presently used in many breast and uterine carcinoma clinical trials.

- *Antiestrogen drugs*, such as tamoxifen and the newer toremifene and raloxifene, block estrogen binding to receptors and estrone sulfate conversion into the active estradiol hormone. Antiestrogens can also inhibit the breast carcinoma growth factor, protein kinase C, and prevent multidrug resistance caused by P-glycoprotein. Because tamoxifen also has proestrogen activity, its use in breast carcinoma may increase the risk of uterine carcinoma.
- *Progesterones with antiestrogen activity*, such as megestrol and medroxyprogesterone, block estrogen receptors and kill cancer cells directly. Progesterones also decrease hormone production by the adrenal gland, increase hormone breakdown, and change tumor handling of hormones. Progesterones prevent menopausal symptoms caused by antiestrogens and improve poor appetite and emaciation.
- *Aromatase inhibitors*, such as letrozole, anastrozole and exemestane, block estrogen production by the adrenal gland. Aromatase inhibitors prevent androgen conversion into estrogen by the cytochrome P450 aromatase enzyme. This is equivalent to "medical removal" of the adrenal gland, which is the sole source of estrogen in postmenopausal patients with breast carcinoma.
- *Synthetic androgens*, such as fluoxymesterone, treat breast carcinoma that has failed other hormone therapies and improve poor appetite and emaciation.
- *Potent estrogens*, such as diethylstilbestrol and estradiol, sometimes work for hormone-sensitive postmenopausal breast carcinoma that has failed other hormone therapies.
- *Compounds structurally similar to the gonadotropin-releasing hormone (analogues)*, such as goserelin and leuprolide, bind receptors better than the hormone to turn off estrogen and progesterone production by the ovary to postmenopausal levels.

Androgen-blocking Therapy.   Androgens made by the testes are the growth factors of normal prostate cells, and prostate cancer cells that secrete the prostate-specific antigen (PSA). Androgen-blockage therapy is presently used in many prostate carcinoma clinical trials. Methods include:

- withdrawing androgens from the body by surgical removal of both testes.
- using analogues of the gonadotropin-releasing hormone to turn off testicular testosterone production.
- using steroidal antiandrogens with progesterone activity, such as cyproterone and megestrol acetate, to block terosterone binding to receptors.
- using nonsteroidal antiandrogens such as flutamide, bicalutamide, or nilutamide to block dihydrotestosterone binding to receptors.
- using the antiandrogen 5-αreductase enzyme inhibitor finasteride, blocks testosterone conversion into the more potent dihydrotestosterone.
- using aminoglutethimide drugs, such as the antifungal agent ketoconazole, to inhibit androgen production by the adrenal gland and testes and to prevent androgen conversion into estrogen by the cytochrome P450 aromatase enzyme.
- using corticosteroid hormones such as hydrocortisone and prednisone, which have considerable anticancer activity.
- using potent estrogens such as diethylstilbestrol and estradiol, which may work in prostate carcinoma.

Somatostatin-blocking Therapy.   Somatostatin is a hormone secreted by carcinoid tumor and pancreatic islet cell carcinoma. It may cause uncomfortable symptoms such as flushing, itching, asthma, palpitation, low blood pressure, diarrhea, and scarring of the heart. Symptomatic tumors may be controlled with the somatostatin analogue octreotide, which binds to the somatostatin receptor better than somatostatin, to block somatostatin activity.

Bone Marrow or Peripheral Stem Cell Transplant

Candidate Malignancies. Transplant is now first-line therapy for high-risk leukemia, which includes Philadelphia chromosome-positive acute lymphoblastic leukemia, acute myelogenous leukemia, chronic myelogenous leukemia, multiple myeloma, myelodysplastic syndromes, poor-biology advanced neuroblastoma, and adult acute lymphoblastic leukemia and chronic lymphocytic leukemia. It is second-line therapy for relapsed or refractory malignancies such as leukemia, lymphoma, histiocytic syndromes, multiple myeloma, Ewing sarcoma, rhabdomyosarcoma, Wilms tumor, retinoblastoma, germ cell, testicular, and brain tumors, and small cell lung, ovarian, renal cell, and breast cancers.

Basic Principles. The whole purpose of the transplant is to allow the use of high doses of chemotherapy and/or total body radiation that would normally destroy bone marrow stem cells, by rescuing the patient with transfused stem cells to repopulate the bone marrow. The bone marrow starts to recover in two to four weeks, but full recovery of blood counts takes months, and normalization of the immune system takes years. Until the blood counts start recovering, transplant patients are kept in isolation. The conditioning regimen used to prepare for transplant is high doses of chemotherapy that mainly has bone marrow rather than organ toxicity. Conditioning regimens include alkylating agents such as busulfan or cyclophosphamide, podophyllotoxins such as etoposide, and platinum compounds such as carboplatin. Transplant is performed when there is only minimal disease remaining after chemotherapy, surgery, and/or radiation. It is contraindicated for progressive disease or cancers unresponsive to chemotherapy.

Rationale. Both previously frozen "committed" and "uncommitted" stem cells are transfused into the patient during transplant. Committed erythroid stem cells make red blood cells, myeloid stem cells make white blood cells, and megakaryocytic stem cells make platelets. Uncommitted stem cells can differentiate into erythroid, myeloid, or megakaryocytic stem cells. Stem cells can be found in both bone marrow and peripheral blood. Bone marrow stem cells can be harvested only by doing hundreds of painful bone marrow aspirates under general anesthesia. Peripheral blood stem cells are harvested by apheresis, a dialysislike process, during the postchemotherapy recovery phase stimulated with a hormone-like compound that promotes neutrophil (granulocyte) production (granulocyte colony-stimulating factor or G-CSF). Peripheral blood stem cell transplant has virtually replaced bone marrow transplant. Since stem cells carry the CD34 marker, anti-CD34 antibody may be used to enrich the stem cell harvest before freezing. Transplants may be from self (autologous) or from others (allogeneic). Allogeneic transplants are from human-leukocyte antigen (HLA) matched sibling or relative donors, or from matched unrelated donors. HLA matching is done by cross-matching white blood cell antigens, analogous to cross-matching ABO and Rh red blood cell groups for blood transfusions.

Autologous Transplant. Using a patient's own stem cells to repopulate the bone marrow only works if it contains no tumor cells. Therefore, stem cell collections may be put through chemical or mechanical removal of tumor cells (purging) before freezing. One method uses a magnet to pull out CD34 stem cells that have reacted with anti-CD34 antibody attached to magnetic beads. This works only if the cancer cells are CD34-negative. Another method uses drugs such as 4-hydroxycyclophosphamide, or antibodies such as the anti-CD20 antibody rituximab, to clean up the stem cell collection.

Autologous peripheral blood stem cell transplant has many advantages: There is no need to find a suitable donor. Peripheral blood stem cell collections are less likely to be contaminated by metastatic tumor cells. Bone marrow recovery is faster, so there is less likelihood of life-threatening bacterial, fungal, and viral infections. There is no risk of developing an Epstein-Barr virus infection that acts like a lymphoid malignancy (lymphoproliferative disease). The secondary cancer risk is lower. The long-term complications of allogeneic transplant are avoided. Such complications include small blood vessel blockage damaging the liver and kidneys (veno-occlusive disease), chronic damage to the lungs, and the graft-versus-host disease described below.

Allogeneic Transplant.   HLA-matched donors may be siblings, relatives, or unrelated donors with the same HLA types. HLA-typing requires a 6/6 match of the major leukocyte histocompatibility antigens. Identical twins, of course, are always 6/6 HLA matches. Full siblings are 6/6 HLA matches in 25 percent of cases, but parents and offspring are rarely 6/6 HLA matches. A 6/6 HLA-matched unrelated donor may also be found through a bone marrow registry search. Allogeneic transplants from 6/6 major histocompatibility antigen-matched donors are often complicated by graft rejection and graft-versus-host disease due to minor histocompatibility antigen mismatches. Graft rejection is caused by recipient T cells rejecting donor stem cells. Graft-versus-host disease is caused by donor CD8 and CD4 T cells and natural killer cells destroying recipient liver, bowel, and skin cells and rejecting bone marrow cells. Removal of donor T cells from the harvested stem cells and treatment with immunosuppressive drugs may reduce the risk of graft-versus-host disease. The major advantage of allogeneic transplant is the graft-versus-cancer phenomenon, in which activated donor T cells help kill the tumor cells in the recipient.

Matched Unrelated Donor Transplant. The possibility of finding a 6/6 HLA-matched unrelated donor through a bone marrow registry search is 70 percent for Caucasians, but much lower for other ethnic groups that are not as well represented in bone marrow registries. Graft-versus-host disease is more likely and more severe from matched unrelated donor transplant because of a higher number of minor histocompatibility antigen mismatches. Nowadays molecular testing allows better matching of minor histocompatibility antigens, reducing the risk of severe graft-versus-host disease.

Mismatched Related Donor Transplant. If no matched related or unrelated donor is available, a relative with 50 percent match of the major histocompatibility antigens (haploid-identical) may be used as the donor. Graft-versus-host disease is very common and severe in such transplants. Despite removal of the T cell from the harvested donor stem cells and more intensive immunosuppression, patients often develop severe graft-versus-host disease and die of life-threatening infections. One possible solution is to render the donor T cells incapable of responding immunologically (anergic), so that they will not react with the recipient antigens.

Cord Blood Transplant. Cord blood contains primitive stem cells that divide very well. Only small numbers of such stem cells are needed to repopulate a destroyed bone marrow. The best response occurs with 6/6 HLA matches. However,

5/6 HLA matches may be used; because cord blood T cells are immature, graft-versus-host disease is rare and less severe.

Supportive Therapy

Basic Principles. Patients can receive cancer therapy only as long as they tolerate the side effects. Therefore, supportive therapy is important because it reduces the complications from treatment. Supportive therapy improves the quality of life of patients during treatment and may mean the difference between cure or failure of treatment. It helps allay the fears of patients, especially if potential complications are explained beforehand.

Management of Short-term Complications

Nausea and Vomiting. Potent antiemetic drugs now available, to prevent nausea and vomiting from drugs such as cisplatin, mechlorethamine, and doxorubicin, block serotonin and 5-hydroxytryptamine receptors in the brain, bowels, and inner ear. These include the 5-hydroxytryptamine blockers ondansetron and granisetron, the serotonin blocker metoclopamide, the cannabinoid compounds marijuana and nabilone, and the potent steroid dexamethasone.

Poor Appetite and Weight Loss. Cancer can cause poor appetite, weight loss, muscle wasting, and emaciation by changing the metabolism of the body through release of cytokines such as tumor necrosis factor and interleukin-6. This may be prevented by the progestogens medroxyprogesterone and megestrol, fish-oil derivatives eicosanoids, melatonin, or thalidomide. Intravenous or nasogastric and gastrostomy feeding may provide temporary nutritional support.

Pain. "Pain teams" are now available in most cancer treatment centers to advise on the types of drugs and routes of administration for different types of pain. The main drugs used are nonopioids, opioids, and adjuvant drugs. Nonopioids include acetaminophen, aspirin, and nonsteroidal anti-inflammatory drugs (NSAIDs). NSAIDs include ibuprofen and naproxen, which block prostaglandin E_2 release in tissue injury. NSAIDs also include the cyclooxygenase-2 enzyme inhibitors celecoxib (Celebrex) and rofecoxib (Vioxx), but these are presently under investigation for possibly increasing the risk of heart attacks. Opioids include codeine, dihydrocodeine, oxycodone, morphine, hydromorphone, methadone, meperidine, and fentanyl. Adjuvant drugs for nerve pain include antidepressants like amitriptyline, anticonvulsants like gabapentin, steroids like dexamethasone, benzodiazepines like clonazepam, local anesthetics like lidocaine, and nerve blockers like alcohol and phenol. Bone pain due to metastasis or osteoporosis may be treated with bisphosphonates like pamidronate, chemotherapy like doxorubicin, calcitonin, gallium nitrate, [89]strontium, and radiation. Pain may also be treated with electric nerve stimulation, acupuncture, heat or cold therapy, and cutting the posterior spinal nerve roots.

Anemia. Anemia is treated with red cell transfusions, using cytomegalovirus-free and radiated blood products to prevent viral infection and graft-versus-host disease from donor T cells engrafting in immunosuppressed patients. Other treatments for anemia include the erythropoietin growth factor to stimulate red cell production, and blood substitutes like hemogloblin-based oxygen carrier, perfluorocarbon emulsion, and liposome-encapsulated hemoglobin.

Bleeding. Bleeding is treated with platelet transfusions, which can be HLA-matched and concentrated for patients that respond poorly to platelets. Other treatments for low platelets include growth factors to stimulate platelet production, such as granulocyte-macrophage colony-stimulating factor (GM-CSF), interleukin-11, and thrombopoietin. Patients with low platelets must avoid drugs that affect clotting, such as aspirin, NSAIDs, Coumadin, and asparaginase chemotherapy.

Fever and Neutropenia.   Patients with low white blood neutrophil count (neutropenia) often develop bacteria and fungal sepsis, or fever of unknown origin. They must be admitted for intravenous broad-spectrum antibiotic therapy. Infectious deaths are now rare because potent antibiotic and antifungal drugs are available. The granulocyte colony-stimulating factor (G-CSF) may reduce the duration of neutropenia, but white cell transfusions are ineffective and dangerous.

Alopecia.   Hair loss from chemotherapy is short-term, but hair loss from radiation is permanent. For cancers with low risk of metastases, hair loss from chemotherapy may be reduced by using an ice cap and applying intermittent pressure to the scalp with a narrow blood pressure cuff during chemotherapy.

Mouth Ulcers and Dental Problems.   Radiation and doxorubicin, daunorubicin, dactinomycin, methotrexate, idarubicin, epirubicin, mitoxantrone, and 5-fluorouracil chemotherapy may cause severe mouth ulcers. They can be treated with benzydamine or betamethasone mouthwashes; prostaglandin E_2 and vitamins E, C, and A to promote healing; sucralfate to provide a protective barrier; chlorhexidine to treat bacterial infection; acyclovir to treat herpes virus infection; nystatin or ketoconazole to treat fungal infections; lidocaine; the chili-pepper extract capsaicin; ice therapy and laser therapy for local pain control; and morphine or fentanyl for systemic pain control.

Radiation Skin and Mucosal Burns.   Modern radiation techniques cause less skin and mucosal burns, especially if anthracycline and dactinomycin chemotherapy and radiosen-sitizing skin applications are avoided. Amifostine may prevent tissue damage by destroying the reactive free radicals released by radiation or chemotherapy. Skin burns may be treated with steroid skin applications. Patients with mucosal burns are sup-ported with intravenous feeding and pain medications. Burns in the mouth may be reduced by good oral hygiene. Burns in the esophagus may be treated with antacids. Burns in the bowels may be reduced by low-residue diet.

Venous Access. Use of central venous lines for blood-taking, chemotherapy, antibiotic, hydration, and blood product therapy is a major advance, particularly for children. Their skin may be numbed with a topical anesthetic to allay the fear of needles.

Management of Long-term Complications. Nowadays, long-term follow-up clinics are set up to provide rehabilita-tion, counseling, and support of patients with therapy-related problems as described in table 5.2 of chapter 5. Discussion about potential therapy-related secondary leukemia or cancer is important for ensuring early diagnosis and timely treatment of such complications.

Alternative Therapy and Complementary Therapy

Focus of Alternative and Complementary Therapy. The National Institutes of Health Office of Alternative Medicine defines complementary and alternative medicine (CAM) as: "a broad domain of healing resources that encompasses all health systems, modalities, and practices and their accompa-nying theories and beliefs, other than those intrinsic to the politically dominant health system of a particular society or culture in a given historical period. CAM includes all such practices and ideas self-defined by their users as preventing or treating illness or promoting health and well-being. Boundaries within CAM and between the CAM domain and the domain of the dominant system are not always sharp or fixed." Briefly, alternative therapy is used instead of conventional therapy, while complementary therapy is used to supplement conventional therapy. Both focus on promoting well-being, treating symptoms, improving general health, and stimulating the immune system. Such therapies have not been tested in clinical trials or have been shown to be ineffective on testing, but are widely used by patients with cancer. Therefore, oncologists should encourage open communication with patients regarding their complementary therapy, to ensure that toxic drugs are not used and interaction with chemotherapy is avoided.

Types of Alternative and Complementary Therapy. The many types of therapy are beyond the scope of this chapter. They include megavitamins such as vitamin C, herb and animal products such as Essiac, mistletoe and shark cartilage, metabolic therapy such as macrobiotic diets, drugs such as Laetrile, antineoplastons and hydrazine sulfate, immune modifiers such as mushroom extracts and thymus therapy, electromagnetism such as therapeutic touch, manipulative therapy such as acupuncture, and supportive therapy such as hypnosis.

Toxicity and Drug Interactions. Most oncology pharmacies now keep a list of drugs with reported toxicities and drug interactions. Some examples include kombucha tea causing cardiac arrest, skullcap causing liver toxicity, chaparral causing hepatitis and liver failure, licorice causing high blood pressure and low serum potassium, garlic decreasing platelet function and potentiating the anticoagulant coumarin, ginger causing clotting problems, ginkgo decreasing platelet function, ginseng interfering with platelet function and reducing coumarin activity, and arnica potentiating coumarin therapy.

Information Sources.   The National Institutes of Health Office of Alternative Medicine and the National Cancer Institute have investigated promising case reports by initiated clinical trials to define objective responses. Information may be obtained from these websites.

- Office of Technology Assessment Report of the Unconventional Cancer Treatments Panel, http://jya.com/otapub.html
- American Cancer Society, www.cancer.org
- National Institutes of Health National Center for Complementary and Alternative Medicine (NCCAM), http://nccam.nih.gov
- National Cancer Institute Office of Cancer Complementary and Alternative Research (OCCAM) http://www.cancer.gov/cam

Palliative Therapy

Purpose.   The purpose of palliative therapy is to support patients when surgery is no longer possible and chemotherapy and radiation have failed to cure their cancers. Aggressive measures that cause pain and complications are avoided, and only acute symptoms are treated. The aim is to improve the quality of life and reduce interventions. Many patients also decide on an order for no cardiopulmonary resuscitation or "do not resuscitate." Parents of children with cancer act as surrogate decision makers to define the level of treatment. Cancer centers have outreach palliative care programs to provide care in the home or at a hospice.

Palliative Measures.   Treatments for poor appetite, weight loss, nausea, pain, anemia, bleeding, fever, and infections have

Table 6.1 Summary of Biological Therapies and How They Work

Subclasses	Mechanisms of Action	Drugs and Agents	Diseases Treated
Immunotherapy	interferons	IFN-α	Kaposi sarcoma, carcinoid, melanoma, bladder and renal cell carcinoma, non-Hodgkin lymphoma, hairy cell and chronic myelogenous leukemia
		IFN-α and retinoic acid	cervix, renal cell, and airway and gastrointestinal carcinoma
		IFN-α and chemotherapy, IL-2, tamoxifen, or steroids	malignant melanoma and non-Hodgkin lymphoma
		IFN-γ	renal cell carcinoma
		IFN-γ and chemotherapy or vaccines	neuroblastoma, malignant melanoma
	interleukins	IL-2 and lymphokine-activated killer cells	non-Hodgkin and Hodgkin lymphoma, melanoma, and renal cell, non–small cell lung, colorectal, and ovarian carcinoma
		IL-2 and tumor-infiltrating lymphocytes, monoclonal antibody, vaccines, or chemotherapy	metastatic melanoma and renal cell carcinoma
	monoclonal antibodies	antibody-dependent cellular cytotoxicity with anti-CD20 antibody (rituximab), anti-HER2/neu antibody (trastuzumab), and anti-GD2 and anti-GD3 antibodies	CD20-positive B-cell lymphoma, leukemia and multiple myeloma, HER2/neu-positive breast carcinoma, GD2-positive neuroblastoma and GD3-positive melanoma

	bispecific monoclonal antibody such as 2B1	HER2/neu-positive breast cancer
	immunocytokine with an antibody fused with IL-2	refractory cancers
	antigrowth factor receptor antibody such as the antiepidermal growth factor receptor MAB225 antibody	epidermal growth factor receptor-positive breast, prostate, head-and-neck, and non–small cell lung carcinoma
	anti-idiotype antibody such as the anti-CD52 Campath-1 antibody	CD52-positive melanoma, colorectal carcinoma, B-cell lymphoma, and leukemia
	radioimmunoconjugate such as the ^{131}iodine/anti-CD20 antibody	CD20-positive B-cell lymphoma and leukemia
	immunotoxin such as the ricin A chain/CD22 antibody	CD22-positive B-cell lymphoma
	chemoconjugate such as the doxorubicin/BR96 antibody	
vaccines	cancer vaccines	refractory leukemia and cancer
		melanoma, follicular lymphoma, and prostate, cervix, non–small cell lung, renal cell, and colon carcinoma
	cancer prevention vaccines	hepatitis B–induced liver cancer, papillomavirus-induced cervix cancer
Hormonal therapy	estrogen-blocking therapy	(1) antiestrogens such as tamoxifen, toremifene, and raloxifene	breast and uterine carcinoma

(Continued)

Table 6.1 (*Continued*)

Subclasses	Mechanisms of Action	Drugs and Agents	Diseases Treated
		(2) progesterones such as megestrol and medroxyprogesterone	
		(3) aromatase inhibitors such as letrozole, anastrozole, and exemestane	
		(4) synthetic androgen such as fluoxymesterone	
		(5) potent estrogens such as estradiol and diethylstilbestrol	
		(6) gonadotropin-releasing hormone analogues such as goserelin and leuprolide	
	androgen-blocking therapy	(1) surgical removal of both testes	prostate carcinoma
		(2) gonadotropin-releasing hormone analogues such as goserelin and leuprolide	
		(3) steroidal antiandrogens such as cyproterone and megestrol acetate	
		(4) nonsteroidal antiandrogens such as flutamide, bicalutamide, and nilutamide	

(Continued)

(5) antiandrogen 5α-reductase enzyme inhibitors such as finasteride

(6) aminoglutethimides such as the antifungal ketoconazole

(7) corticosteroids such as hydrocortisone and prednisone

(8) estrogen therapy such as diethylstilbestrol and estradiol

	somatostatin analogue octreotide	somatostatin-blocking therapy	somatostatin-secreting carcinoid tumor and pancreatic islet cell carcinoma
Bone marrow or peripheral stem cell transplant	rescue bone marrow after lethal chemotherapy and/or total body radiation	autologous, allogeneic, matched-unrelated, cord blood, and mismatched related donor transplant	First-line therapy for high-risk leukemia, multiple myeloma, myelodysplastic syndromes, poor-biology advanced neuroblastoma; second-line therapy for relapsed or refractory leukemia, lymphoma, histiocytic syndromes, multiple myeloma, Ewing sarcoma, rhabdomyosarcoma, Wilms tumor, retinoblastoma, germ cell, testicular and brain tumors, and small cell lung, ovarian, renal cell, and breast cancers

Table 6.1 (*Continued*)

Subclasses	Mechanisms of Action	Drugs and Agents	Diseases Treated
Supportive therapy	short-term complications	venous access, treatment of nausea and vomiting, poor appetite and weight loss, pain, anemia, bleeding, fever and neutropenia, infections, mouth ulcers and dental problems, hair loss, and radiation skin and mucosal damage	relevant for all cancers
	long-term complications	rehabilitation, counseling, and treatment of therapy-related problems; alert patients to early diagnosis and timely treatment of secondary cancers	
Alternative and complementary therapy	nonconventional therapy	aim at treating cancer, and improving general well-being and immune system	anecdotal treatment of unproven efficacy for cancer
Palliative therapy	provide comfort measures	symptomatic treatment for weight loss, pain, anemia, bleeding, fever, infections	relevant for all cancers

been discussed in the supportive therapy section; however, the indications become different in these cases. For example, patients may elect not to have blood and platelet transfusions, or antibiotic therapy, unless they become symptomatic. Poor appetite and weight loss are treated with hydration rather than attempts to improve nutrition. Pain and nausea and vomiting are treated aggressively to maintain a good quality of life.

7. Therapies for Childhood Cancer

Important advances in combination therapy have made most childhood cancers curable. Chemotherapy forms the backbone of combination therapy. Two mandates in childhood cancer therapy for decreasing long-term morbidity are avoiding radiation and reducing treatment.

Issues in Treatment of Childhood Cancers

Importance of Avoiding Radiation. Combination therapy means chemotherapy to reduce the tumor load, followed by "cancer surgery"—removing the remaining tumor and adjacent involved structures in one piece to achieve negative surgical margins free of tumor cells microscopically. Total removal is not possible if vital organs are involved, the cancer is no longer localized to one location, or the surgery is too mutilating. The goal of total resection is to avoid radiation. Radiation causes more lasting side effects in children than in adults. The younger the children, the more severe are the anatomical, cosmetic, functional, and intellectual consequences of radiation. Radiation also causes an about 5–15 percent lifelong risk of secondary cancers within the radiation field; in some childhood cancers, such as hereditary retinoblastoma, the lifelong risk is even greater.

Importance of Reducing Therapy. In diseases where cure rates approach 100 percent, the goal is to reduce therapy to decrease short-term and long-term morbidity. Each cancer may now be classified by pathology and biology as favorable or unfavorable. For favorable disease, therapy may be reduced and treatment shortened. This decreases the risk of acute chemotherapy complications, such as life-threatening infection when all the blood counts are low (pancytopenia). For example, localized and favorable Wilms tumor is now treated with removal of the kidney (nephrectomy) without radiation, and chemotherapy has been shortened from years to weeks. Favorable acute lymphoblastic leukemia is now treated with three- instead of five-year chemotherapy, with no brain and spinal cord radiation that causes lasting intellectual and learning problems, short stature, growth hormone or thyroid deficiency, and, rarely, malignant brain tumors. Instead, methotrexate, cytarabine, and hydrocortisone are given by lumbar puncture (intrathecally), and intravenous high-dose methotrexate has been substituted to prevent central nervous system leukemia.

The Twelve Most Common Cancers in Children. The twelve most common childhood cancers according to frequency are: leukemia, lymphoma, brain and spinal cord tumors, lymphoma, neuroblastoma, soft tissue sarcoma, Wilms tumor, bone sarcoma, retinoblastoma, germ cell tumors, hepatoblastoma, melanoma, and carcinoma of the thyroid, salivary glands, nasopharynx, colon, and pancreas. Childhood cancers differ from adult cancers in types, pathology, biology, treatment, and cure rates.

Pathology Differences Between Childhood and Adult Cancers. Children develop fetuslike and embryolike (embryonal), blood-forming (hematologic), or lymphocyte-forming (lymphatic) tumors, while adults predominantly develop carcinoma of different organs or tissues. The most common childhood cancers are embryonal in origin, resembling immature (undifferentiated) tissues in fetuses and embryos, which retain the potential to branch out and develop into different types of mature tissues. Embryonal tumors include medulloblastoma that arises from neural tissue of the brain, neuroblastoma from neural tissue in the periphery nerve ganglia or adrenal medulla, Wilms tumor in kidney, retinoblastoma from the retina, germ cell tumor mostly in the ovary and testis, hepatoblastoma in the liver, and soft tissue and bone sarcoma from the middle embryonic cell layer (mesoderm or mesenchyme). Leukemia and lymphoma arise from immature or mature precursor cells (stem cells) that ultimately develop into red blood cells, white blood cells and platelets in the bone marrow, and lymphoid cells in the thymus glands and lymphatic tissues. Carcinomas are rare in children but, when they occur, are no different in type, location, and behavior from their adult counterparts.

Differences in Chemotherapy Response Between Childhood and Adult Cancers.   Because they arise from undifferentiated tissues that are highly responsive to chemotherapy, most childhood malignancies, such as embryonal and mesenchymal tumors, leukemia, and lymphoma, can be cured Adult malignancies, such as carcinomas, arise from more mature tissues that generally respond poorly to chemotherapy.

Biologic Differences Between Childhood and Adult Cancers. The biology of a cancer determines its aggressiveness and response to therapy. Essentially, cancers arise (carcinogenesis) because of genetic mistakes (mutations) made during normal cell division. A mutation may be acquired in an oncogene or a tumor suppressor gene. One oncogene mutation is enough to initiate cancer, but two tumor suppressor mutations are required for carcinogenesis. The first mutation occurs on one arm of a chromosome (allele), causing the two tumor suppressor genes on the two alleles to become different, or acquiring heterozygosity. When a second mutation occurs on the other allele, both tumor suppressor genes on the two alleles now become different (loss of heterozygosity).

After cancer initiates, its progression depends on acquiring further oncogene mutations or tumor suppressor gene mutations. When mutations result in multiple copies of an oncogene (amplification), proliferation, invasion, and spread of cancer cells are switched on. When mutations result in loss or deactivation of a tumor suppressor gene, division, differentiation, and death of cancer cells become deregulated. Other mutations may cause resistance to drugs or radiation. Acquiring unfavorable mutations confers poor biology that makes cancers more aggressive, less sensitive to treatment, and more difficult to cure. Poor biology generally goes with advanced stages, favorable biology with early stages. In general, adult cancers tend to have poorer biology, having acquired more unfavorable mutations than childhood cancers.

Biologic Differences Between Childhood and Adult Leukemia and Lymphoma. In general, childhood leukemia and lymphoma originate from less mature hematopoietic and lymphoid cells than do their adult counterparts. Children tend to have acute leukemia and lymphoma, whereas adults usually have chronic forms of these diseases. Acute leukemia and lymphoma are so-called because death occurs in days to weeks if untreated, whereas chronic leukemia and lymphoma are so-called since death occurs slowly over months to years. Acute lymphoblastic leukemia is the most common leukemia in children. Acute myelogenous leukemia and chronic myelogenous leukemia are less common, but chronic lymphocytic leukemia is never seen in childhood. In general, acute leukemia and lymphoma respond much better to chemotherapy than chronic forms of these diseases. Cure rates are much higher for acute than for chronic leukemia and lymphoma.

Acute lymphoblastic leukemia is also easier to cure than acute myelogenous leukemia. Chronic myelogenous leukemia is now curable with new molecular targeted therapy (see chapter 9), chemotherapy, and bone marrow transplant. Chronic lymphocytic leukemia affects older patients and does not respond to chemotherapy, but its course is indolent, allowing patients to live for years without treatment, often ultimately dying of unrelated causes. Childhood acute lymphomas respond well to chemotherapy because the cells are immature and rapidly dividing. Adult chronic lymphomas respond poorly to chemotherapy because the cells are mature and divide slowly. These chronic lymphomas are called "low-grade"; although they may be controlled for years with surgery and radiation, they ultimately cause death of the patients. Overall, children do better and have higher cure rates than adults when they have the same types of leukemia or lymphoma. This is probably related to other, as yet undefined unfavorable biological factors in adult leukemia and lymphoma.

Biologic Differences Between Childhood and Adult Sarcoma. Childhood soft tissue sarcoma differs from adult sarcoma. Children commonly have embryonal rhabdomyosarcoma, which arises from immature cells resembling embryo and fetal muscle cells and is chemosensitive and curable. Adults generally have alveolar or pleomorphic forms of rhabdomyosarcoma, which arise from more mature mesenchymal tissues and are aggressive and resistant to chemotherapy, with widespread disease at presentation. Children also have sarcoma arising from the bone (osteosarcoma) and the periosteum that covers the bone (Ewing sarcoma, Ewing-like primitive peripheral neuroectodermal tumor or PNET). The cure rates of such tumors are better in children than in adults because childhood sarcomas are generally more responsive to chemotherapy. Adults have the rarer sarcomas arising from cartilage (chondrosarcoma), which responds poorly to chemotherapy.

Undifferentiated Childhood Cancers with Poor Prognosis. Some immature childhood tumors respond to chemotherapy initially but recur despite intensive therapy that includes surgery, radiation, and bone marrow transplant. One example is neuroblastoma that has poor biology and has spread at diagnosis. Poor biology in neuroblastoma is due to acquiring oncogene mutations, such as *MYCN* gene amplification, and tumor suppressor gene mutations, such as chromosome 1p deletion.

Principles of Treatment of Childhood Cancers

General Principles.   Children with cancer are generally treated on clinical trials, or with standard regimens if no clinical trials are open, under the auspices of a pediatric cooperative called the Children's Oncology Group in the U.S., Canada, and some European and South American centers. Chemotherapy protocols consist of several drugs (combination chemotherapy). Each block of chemotherapy drugs is called a cycle. Each cycle is usually three weeks apart. Treatment usually lasts for about a year. Most protocols are intensive, with drug doses that cause severe pancytopenia, in which red blood cell counts, white blood cell counts, and platelet counts become very low but recover before the next cycle. Children are carefully supported during pancytopenia and immunosuppression, as described in chapter 6. Drug doses are calculated to avoid severe and irreversible damage to the kidneys, liver, brain, nerves, hearing, and bowel lining. Treatment at diagnosis is called first-line therapy. Treatment at relapse is called salvage therapy, using second- or third-line protocols. Because present-day first-line therapy is very intensive, salvage therapy is generally not curative, although it may prolong survival.

Curability of the Twelve Most Common Childhood Cancers. About eleven out of 100,000 children develop cancer every year in the United States. Table 7.1 summarizes the twelve most common cancers by annual incidence, order of frequency, and primary and relapse therapy. The annual incidence is the number of new diagnoses in every 100,000 children each year. The treatment results are expressed as overall five-year cure rates. The five-year cure rates are also quoted separately for "good-risk" and "poor-risk" disease. Cancers are generally classified as local disease confined to organ of origin (Stage I), regional disease involving adjacent tissues (Stage II), extensive disease (Stage III), and distant metastases (Stage IV). Good-risk disease generally means Stages I and II with favorable biology, whereas poor-risk disease means Stages III and IV with unfavorable biology. Most good-risk disease is curable. Many instances of poor-risk disease are also curable but require more intensive therapy. Curable malignancies include leukemia (acute lymphoblastic and myelogenous, chronic myelogenous), lymphoma (Hodgkin and non-Hodgkin), germ cell tumors, Wilms tumor, retinoblastoma, soft tissue sarcoma (embryonal and undifferentiated rhabdomyosarcoma), bone sarcoma (osteosarcoma, Ewing sarcoma, primitive peripheral neuroectodermal tumor or PNET), medulloblastoma, and some cases of neuroblastoma.

Primary and Second-Line Chemotherapy. A full description of the chemotherapy protocols is beyond the scope of this book, but table 7.2 provides a brief summary of those malignancies in which chemotherapy plays a major role as primary or second-line therapy. Primary therapy for childhood cancers is generally chemotherapy and surgery, since most cancers are

Table 7.1 Summary of the Twelve Most Common Childhood Cancers and Treatment Outcomes

Rank	Annual Incidence	Subtypes	Primary Therapies	Relapse Therapies	Five-Year Cure Rates
#1	**Leukemia: 3.02/100,000 children/year**				
	Acute lymphoblastic leukemia: 1.76/100,000 children/year	(1) Burkitt, precursor and common B-cell (2) lymphoblastic T-cell (3) biphenotypic: lymphoblastic myelogenous	(1) chemotherapy (2) CNS prophylaxis: intrathecal drugs, high-dose methotrexate, or brain radiation	(1) chemotherapy (2) alloBMT (3) radiation	80% overall 70% poor-risk 90% good-risk
	Acute undifferentiated leukemia: 0.66/100,000 children/year		(1) chemotherapy (2) CNS prophylaxis: intrathecal drugs, high-dose methotrexate, or brain radiation	(1) chemotherapy (2) alloBMT (3) radiation	60% overall 50% poor-risk 70% good-risk
	Acute myelogenous leukemia (0.51/100,000 children/year)	M0, undifferentiated; M1, poorly differentiated; M2, M3, differentiated; M4, myelomonoblastic; M5, monoblastic; M6, erythroblastic; M7, megakaryoblastic	(1) chemotherapy (2) CNS prophylaxis: intrathecal chemotherapy (3) auto/alloBMT	(1) chemotherapy (2) 2nd alloBMT	50% overall 40% poor-risk 60% good-risk

(*Continued*)

Table 7.1 (*Continued*)

Rank	Annual Incidence	Subtypes	Primary Therapies	Relapse Therapies	Five-Year Cure Rates
	Chronic myelogenous leukemia (0.09/100,000 children/year)	(1) adult-type (2) juvenile-type	(1) chemotherapy (2) alloBMT	(1) chemotherapy (2) 2nd alloBMT	50% overall 40% poor-risk 60% good-risk
#2	**Central nervous system tumors (2.12/100,000 children/year)**				
	Brain tumors (2/100,000 children/year)	(1) brain stem or optic nerve glioma, astrocytoma, malignant astrocytoma, glioblastoma multiforme (GBM) (2) ependymoma (3) choroid plexus cancer, craniopharyngioma	(1) surgery (2) radiation (3) chemotherapy	(1) surgery (2) chemotherapy (3) autoBMT for medulloblastoma (4) palliative radiation	medulloblastoma 65% GBM 0% 20–90% overall for other brain tumors
	Spinal tumors (0.12/100,000 children/year)	(1) astrocytoma (2) ependymoma (3) sarcoma, lymphoma, neuroblastoma, chordoma	(1) surgery (2) radiation (3) chemotherapy	(1) surgery (2) chemotherapy (3) palliative radiation	60% overall 50% poor-risk 70% good-risk

#	Category	Types	Treatment	Treatment	Outcome
#3	**Lymphoma and related diseases (1.37/100,000 children/year)**				
	Non-Hodgkin lymphoma (0.7/100,000 children/year)	(1) precursor B-cell, Burkitt, diffuse large cell (2) precursor T-cell, lymphoblastic, diffuse large cell (3) diffuse null large cell	(1) chemotherapy (2) CNS prophylaxis: intrathecal drugs	(1) chemotherapy (2) auto/alloBMT (3) radiation	80% overall 70% poor-risk 90% good-risk
	Hodgkin lymphoma (0.6/100,000 children/year)	(1) lymphocyte-predominant or rich (2) nodular sclerosis (3) mixed cellularity (4) lymphocyte-depleted (5) unclassifiable	(1) chemotherapy (2) radiation	(1) chemotherapy (2) auto/alloBMT (3) palliative radiation	80% overall 70% poor-risk 90% good-risk
	Histiocytic syndromes (0.07/100,000 children/year)	(1) eosinophilic granuloma (2) Hand-Schüller-Christian disease (3) Letterer-Siwe disease (4) malignant histiocytosis	(1) chemotherapy (2) radiation	(1) chemotherapy (2) auto/alloBMT (3) palliative radiation	70% overall 30% poor-risk 100% good-risk
#4	**Neuroblastoma: 0.81/100,000 children/year**				
	Localized (0.41/100,000 children/year)	(1) neuroblastoma (2) ganglioneuroblastoma (3) ganglioneuroma	surgery	(1) surgery (2) chemotherapy (3) radiation	100% overall

(*Continued*)

Table 7.1 (*Continued*)

Rank	Annual Incidence	Subtypes	Primary Therapies	Relapse Therapies	Five-Year Cure Rates
	Generalized (0.4/100,000 children/year)	(1) unfavorable biology (2) high-stage	(1) chemotherapy (2) surgery (3) radiation (4) auto/alloBMT (5) differentiation: *cis*-retinoic acid	(1) chemotherapy (2) surgery (3) 2nd alloBMT (4) palliative radiation	20% overall 10% poor-risk 30% good-risk
#5	**Soft tissue sarcoma (0.78/100,000 children/year)**				
	Rhabdomyosarcoma (0.38/100,000 children/year)	(1) embryonal (2) alveolar (3) undifferentiated (4) mixed (5) pleomorphic	(1) chemotherapy (2) surgery (3) radiation (4) auto/alloBMT for metastatic	(1) chemotherapy (2) surgery (3) auto/alloBMT (4) palliative radiation	60% overall 20% poor-risk 80% good-risk
	Other sarcoma (0.4/100,000 children/year)	(1) malignant fibrous histiocytoma (2) synovial sarcoma (3) aggressive fibromatosis (4) fibrosarcoma (5) neurogenic sarcoma	(1) surgery (2) radiation (3) chemotherapy, lesser role	(1) chemotherapy (2) surgery (3) palliative radiation	50% overall 20% poor-risk 60% good-risk

#	Category / Type	Treatment	Outcome
#6	**Wilms and renal tumors (0.73/100,000 children/year)**		
	Wilms tumor (0.7/100,000 children/year) (1) classic Wilms (2) anaplastic Wilms (3) unfavorable biology clear cell sarcoma (4) unfavorable biology rhabdoid tumor	(1) surgery (2) chemotherapy (3) radiation	(1) surgery (2) chemotherapy (3) auto/alloBMT (4) palliative radiation → 80% overall, 50% poor-risk, 100% good-risk
	Congenital mesoblastic nephroma CMN (0.02/100,000 children/year) (1) classical CMN (2) aggressive cellular CMN	(1) surgery (2) chemotherapy rarely needed	(1) surgery (2) chemotherapy (3) radiation → 98–100% overall
	Renal cell carcinoma (0.01/100,000 children/year) see adult disease	see adult disease	see adult disease → 60% overall, 5% poor-risk, 70% good-risk
#7	**Bone sarcoma (0.46/100,000 children/year)**		
	Osteosarcoma (0.35/100,000 children/year) (1) osteosarcoma (2) chondrosarcoma	(1) chemotherapy (2) surgery	(1) chemotherapy (2) surgery (3) palliative radiation → 60% overall, 10% poor-risk, 80% good-risk
	Ewing sarcoma (0.11/100,000 children/year) (1) Ewing sarcoma (2) primitive peripheral neuroectodermal tumor (PNET)	(1) surgery (2) chemotherapy (3) radiation (4) auto/alloBMT for metastatic	(1) chemotherapy (2) surgery (3) auto/alloBMT (4) palliative radiation → 50% overall, 10% poor-risk, 70% good-risk

(*Continued*)

Table 7.1 (Continued)

Rank	Annual Incidence	Subtypes	Primary Therapies	Relapse Therapies	Five-Year Cure Rates
#8	**Retinoblastoma (0.34/100,000 children/year)**				
	Retinoblastoma	(1) retinoblastoma (2) benign retinoma (3) medulloepithelioma (very rare)	(1) chemotherapy (2) laser therapy, cryotherapy (3) unilateral: enucleation only (4) bilateral: enucleation if in danger of spreading outside eye	(1) enucleation (2) chemotherapy (3) laser therapy, cryotherapy (4) radioactive plaque (5) radiation (6) auto/alloBMT for metastatic	70% overall 30% poor-risk 100% good-risk
#9	**Germ cell tumors (0.33/100,000 children/year)**				
	Gonadal and nongonadal germ cell tumor	(1) germinoma (2) dysgerminoma (3) embryonal carcinoma (4) endodermal sinus tumor (5) choriocarcinoma (6) malignant teratoma	(1) surgery (2) chemotherapy	(1) chemotherapy (2) surgery (3) radiation (4) auto/alloBMT (5) radiation	80% overall 50% poor-risk 90% good-risk
#10	**Liver tumors (0.08/100,000 children/year)**				
	Hepatoblastoma	(1) embryonal	(1) chemotherapy	(1) chemotherapy	60% overall

(0.07/100,000 children/year)	(2) fetal (3) mixed (4) mesenchymal	(2) surgery (3) liver transplant	(2) surgery (3) liver transplant (4) palliative radiation	20% poor-risk 80% good-risk
Hepatocellular carcinoma (0.01/100,000 children/year)	see adult disease	see adult disease	see adult disease	10% overall 5% poor-risk 15% good-risk

#11 Melanoma and skin cancer (0.08/100,000 children/year)

Malignant melanoma (0.04/100,000 children/year)	see adult disease	see adult disease	see adult disease	70% overall 30% poor-risk 95% good-risk
Other skin cancers (0.04/100,000 children/year)	see adult disease	see adult disease	see adult disease	90% overall 80% poor-risk 100% good-risk

#12 Carcinoma (0.65/100,000 children/year)

Thyroid (0.14/100,000 children/year)	(1) well-differentiated papillary, follicular, Hürthle cell carcinoma (2) anaplastic	(1) surgery (2) ^{131}iodine therapy (3) chemotherapy	(1) surgery (2) palliative radiation (3) chemotherapy (4) preventive diet	90% overall 80% poor-risk 100% good-risk

(Continued)

Table 7.1 (*Continued*)

Rank	Annual Incidence	Subtypes	Primary Therapies	Relapse Therapies	Five-Year Cure Rates
		(3) medullary thyroid cancer (4) lymphoma, sarcoma		(avoid low-iodine; cabbage, shellfish high in iodine)	
	Nasopharynx (0.01/100,000 children/year)	(1) keratinizing squamous cell, nonkeratinizing squamous cell, undifferentiated carcinoma (2) other cancers (lymphoma, juvenile angiofibroma)	(1) surgery (2) radiation (3) chemotherapy	(1) chemotherapy (2) surgery (3) palliative radiation (4) preventive diet (avoid nitrosamine in salt-cured food)	70% overall 60% poor-risk 90% good-risk
	Salivary gland, colon and pancreas cancer (0.5/100,000 children/year)	see adult disease	see adult disease	see adult disease	50% overall 10% poor-risk 90% good-risk

Abbreviations: autoBMT is autologous bone marrow/stem cell transplant; alloBMT is allogeneic bone marrow/stem cell transplant. Result of treatment is measured as estimated five-year cure rate, which means the proportion of patients alive and disease-free five years from diagnosis that likely are cured of cancer. In general, good-risk disease is localized with favorable biology, and poor-risk disease is metastatic with unfavorable biology.

Table 7.2 Primary and Second-Line Chemotherapy for Twelve Common Childhood Cancers

Incidence Rank	Primary Chemotherapy and Other Therapy for Newly Diagnosed Cancers	Second-Line Chemotherapy and Other Therapy for Relapsed Cancers	Death Rank
1	**Leukemia**		6
	Acute lymphoblastic and undifferentiated leukemia:	doxorubicin, mitoxantrone, epirubicin, idarubicin, teniposide, etoposide, vinblastine, vindesine, irinotecan, topotecan, camptothecin	
	(1) *Induction*: prednisone/dexamethasone, vincristine, daunorubicin, asparaginase		
	(2) *Consolidation*: cyclophosphamide, high-dose methotrexate, high-dose cytarabine, doxorubicin, cytarabine, asparaginase		
	(3) *CNS prophylaxis*: cytarabine, methotrexate, hydrocortisone		
	(4) *Maintenance and reinduction*: methotrexate, mercaptopurine, thioguanine, prednisone, vincristine		
	Acute myelogenous and juvenile chronic myelogenous leukemia:	doxorubicin, mitoxantrone, epirubicin, idarubicin, teniposide, etoposide, vindesine, irinotecan, topotecan, camptothecin	
	(1) *Induction*: daunorubicin, cytarabine, high-dose cytarabine		
	(2) *Maintenance*: daunorubicin, cytarabine, high-dose cytarabine, thioguanine		

(Continued)

Table 7.2. (*Continued*)

Incidence Rank	Primary Chemotherapy and Other Therapy for Newly Diagnosed Cancers	Second-Line Chemotherapy and Other Therapy for Relapsed Cancers	Death Rank
	(3) *CNS prophylaxis*: intrathecal cytarabine (4) *Reinduction and maintenance for M3 acute promyelocytic leukemia*: all-*trans*-retinoic acid (ATRA), idarubicin, cytarabine, mitoxantrone, etoposide		
	Chronic myelogenous leukemia: (1) chemotherapy: busulfan, hydroxyurea (2) chemotherapy-biologic therapy: cytarabine with interferon	daunorubicin, doxorubicin, mitoxantrone, idarubicin, epirubicin, high-dose cytarabine, molecular therapy (see chapters 8 and 9), deoxycytidine-inducing DNA demethylation	
2	Medulloblastoma and other brain tumors (1) ICE: ifosfamide, carboplatin, etoposide (2) Other combinations: cisplatin, vincristine, cyclophosphamide, dexamethasone	Mustargen, vincristine, prednisone, procarbazine, vinblastine, lomustine, carmustine	2
3	Lymphoma and related conditions Non-Hodgkin lymphoma: (1) *Induction*: prednisone/dexamethasone, vincristine, doxorubicin, cyclophosphamide	mitoxantrone, epirubicin, idarubicin, teniposide, etoposide, vinblastine, vindesine, irinotecan, topotecan, camptothecin, ifosfamide, carboplatin	7

	(2) *Maintenance:* doxorubicin, high-dose cytarabine, cyclophosphamide, high-dose methotrexate, mercaptopurine, thioguanine (3) *CNS prophylaxis:* cytarabine, methotrexate, hydrocortisone Hodgkin lymphoma: (1) MOPP: Mustargen, vincristine, procarbazine, prednisone (2) COPP: cyclophosphamide, vincristine, procarbazine, prednisone (3) ABVD: doxorubicin, bleomycin, vinblastine, dacarbazine Histiocytic syndromes: prednisone/dexamethasone, etoposide, vincristine	daunorubicin, mitoxantrone, epirubicin, idarubicin, ifosfamide, etoposide, carboplatin, vindesine, irinotecan, topotecan, camptothecin, carboplatin	1
4	**Neuroblastoma** vincristine, doxorubicin, cyclophosphamide, ifosfamide, etoposide, cisplatin, carboplatin	daunorubicin, doxorubicin, cytarabine, high-dose cytarabine, methotrexate, cyclophosphamide, mercaptopurine, thioguanine, ifosfamide, teniposide, carboplatin	4
5	**Rhabdomyosarcoma and other soft tissue sarcoma**	mitoxantrone, epirubicin, idarubicin, teniposide, irinotecan, topotecan, camptothecin, paclitaxel	

(*Continued*)

Table 7.2. (*Continued*)

Incidence Rank	Primary Chemotherapy and Other Therapy for Newly Diagnosed Cancers	Second-Line Chemotherapy and Other Therapy for Relapsed Cancers	Death Rank
	(1) VAC: vincristine, dactinomycin, cyclophosphamide (2) VAdriaC: vincristine, doxorubicin, cyclophosphamide (3) IE: ifosfamide, etoposide	mitoxantrone, epirubicin, idarubicin, teniposide, irinotecan, topotecan, camptothecin, carboplatin	
6	**Wilms tumor, clear cell sarcoma, and rhabdoid tumor** vincristine, doxorubicin, dactinomycin, cyclophosphamide, ifosfamide, etoposide	ifosfamide, teniposide, etoposide, mitoxantrone, epirubicin, idarubicin, irinotecan, topotecan, camptothecin, carboplatin	8
7	**Bone sarcoma** Osteosarcoma: doxorubicin-cisplatin; high-dose methotrexate-leucovorin; IE: ifosfamide, etoposide	(1) chemotherapy: BCD, bleomycin, cyclophosphamide, dactinomycin; epirubicin, mitoxantrone, idarubicin, teniposide, irinotecan, topotecan, camptothecin (2) biologic therapy: interferon, BCG, lung metastases therapy with granulocyte-macrophage colony-stimulating factor (GM-CSF) or muramyltripeptide phosphatidylethanolamine (MTP-PE)	3

Ewing sarcoma, primitive peripheral neuroectodermal tumor (PNET):
(1) VAC: vincristine, dactinomycin, cyclophosphamide
(2) VAdriaC: vincristine, doxorubicin, cyclophosphamide
(3) IE: ifosfamide, etoposide

mitoxantrone, epirubicin, idarubicin, teniposide, irinotecan, topotecan, camptothecin, cisplatin, carboplatin — 12

Retinoblastoma
(1) CEV: carboplatin, etoposide, vincristine
(2) CEV with cyclosporine A: reversal of multidrug resistance

doxorubicin, ifosfamide, teniposide, cyclophosphamide — 9

Germ cell tumors
etoposide, cisplatin/carboplatin, bleomycin, vincristine/vinblastine, ifosfamide

teniposide, vincristine or vinblastine, carboplatin, ifosfamide, cyclophosphamide, doxorubicin, mitoxantrone, epirubicin, idarubicin, irinotecan, topotecan, camptothecin, paclitaxel — 10

Hepatoblastoma and hepatocellular carcinoma
doxorubicin, cisplatin

epirubicin, mitoxantrone, idarubicin, ifosfamide, etoposide, teniposide, carboplatin, vincristine, 5-fluorouracil, lomustine — 5

Malignant melanoma and other skin cancers
see adult disease

see adult disease — 11

(Continued)

Table 7.2 (Continued)

Incidence Rank	Primary Chemotherapy and Other Therapy for Newly Diagnosed Cancers	Second-Line Chemotherapy and Other Therapy for Relapsed Cancers	Death Rank
12	**Carcinoma** Thyroid carcinoma: doxorubicin, dacarbazine, 5-fluorouracil, streptozotocin Nasopharynx carcinoma: (1) CMF: cyclophosphamide, methotrexate, 5-fluorouracil (2) PBF: cisplatin, bleomycin, 5-fluorouracil (3) VAC: vincristine, doxorubicin, cyclophosphamide Colon and pancreas carcinoma: see adult disease	(1) chemotherapy: doxorubicin, cisplatin (2) gene therapy (1) FMEP: 5-fluorouracil, mitomycin C, epirubicin, cisplatin (2) F-BEP: 5-fluorouracil, bleomycin, epirubicin, cisplatin; carboplatin-5-fluorouracil; carboplatin-paclitaxel see adult disease	11

sensitive to chemotherapy. Surgery is often used so that radiation therapy may be avoided, as discussed in chapter 5. Second-line therapy for childhood cancers may consist of alternative chemotherapy, further surgery, radiation, biological therapy, and molecular targeted therapy. Those patients who respond a second time may receive further high-dose consolidation chemotherapy, with marrow rescue by autologous or allogeneic stem cells from the bone marrow, peripheral blood, or cord blood, as described in chapter 6. Because numerous protocols exist, only one or two main examples are included shown in bold, with treatment phases shown in italics (as defined in chapter 1). By far the most common cause of death from childhood cancer is neuroblastoma, closely followed by brain tumor. Death from retinoblastoma is rare since less than 5 percent of cases have spread outside the eye at diagnosis. Deaths from melanoma, skin cancer, and other carcinoma are also rare because these are very rare diseases in children. The order of frequency of deaths is also shown for comparison in table 7.2, but actual death rates are not available for childhood cancers.

Screening for High-risk "Cancer Syndromes." Cancer is more common in children with certain syndromes, and screening ensures early diagnosis. High-risk predisposing conditions exist for almost every type of cancer: (1) leukemia: Downs, Li-Fraumeni (*p53* gene mutation), ataxia-telangietasia, Blooms, Fanconi, and neurofibromatosis type 1 (NF-1) syndromes; (2) brain tumor: Downs, Li-Fraumeni, ataxia-telangietasia, Gorlin, and NF-1 syndromes; (3) lymphoma: ataxia-telangietasia and NF-1 syndromes, HIV infection; (4) neuroblastoma: NF-1, Beckwith-Wiedemann, fetal-alcohol, and fetal-hydantoin syndromes; (5) soft tissue and bone sarcoma: Li-Fraumeni and Beckwith-Wiedemann syndromes, retinoblastoma, previous radiation; (6) Wilms tumor: Beckwith-Wiedemann, hemihypertrophy, aniridia and Denys-Drash syndromes; (7) retinoblastoma: familial and 13q⁻ syndromes; (8) hepatoblastoma: Beckwith-Wiedemann and familial polyposis coli syndromes; (9) thyroid cancer: multiple endocrine neoplasia (MEN 2a or 2b), Gardner and Cowden syndromes, previous radiation; and (10) nasopharynx cancer: Epstein-Barr virus infection, certain high-risk subtypes of white blood cell antigens.

8. Therapies for Cancer in Adults

The philosophy for treatment of cancers in adults is quite different from that for children. This is mainly due to the differences in tumor types, pathology, biology, and sensitivity to chemotherapy.

Issues Related to Treatment of Adult Cancers

The Twenty-Four Most Common Cancers in Adults. The twenty-four most common adult cancers according to frequency are: carcinoma of skin, prostate, breast, lung, colon and uterus, lymphoma, bladder carcinoma, ovarian carcinoma, malignant melanoma, anorectal carcinoma, oropharyngeal carcinoma, leukemia, carcinoma of kidney, pancreas, cervix and stomach, brain and spinal cord tumors, liver and biliary tract carcinoma, multiple myeloma, esophageal carcinoma, soft tissue sarcoma, testicular carcinoma, and bone sarcoma.

Preponderance of Carcinoma in Adults. In adults, the most common form of cancer is carcinoma. Carcinoma is a malignancy of epithelial or endothelial tissues, which are mature and differentiated tissues that lack the potential to branch out to develop into different types of tissues. Because carcinoma is derived from mature tissues, they are relatively insensitive to chemotherapy. Carcinoma may arise from virtually every organ and tissue. It is a cancer of aging tissues—particularly for prostate gland, breast, and colon carcinoma, in which the incidences increase with age. This is because initiation of a carcinoma depends on the accumulation of seven or more mutations in the same cell, which takes time, often several decades. Some mutations may be inherited, but most mutations are acquired through exposure to an agent that can induce mutations (mutagen). Important mutagens include sunlight, tobacco, viruses, toxins, and chemicals. The drugs and radiation used for treatment of cancer are also mutagens.

Adult Cancers Often Respond Poorly to Chemotherapy. Adult cancers are generally not very sensitive to chemotherapy, with few that can be cured by chemotherapy alone. The only chemotherapy-responsive adult malignancies are germ cell tumors (embryonal carcinoma, seminoma, dysgerminoma, choriocarcinoma), acute lymphoblastic and myelogenous leukemia, certain forms of lymphoma, and, rarely, small cell lung and ovarian carcinoma. Even so, adult acute lymphoblastic and myelogenous leukemia require upfront bone marrow or stem cell transplant since the prognosis is poorer than for children. Carcinomas are relatively insensitive to chemotherapy, but there is some response to platinums, camptothecin, taxanes, anthracyclines, anthracenedione, alkylating agents, antimetabolites, mitomycin C, or bleomycin. Good responses, however, are rare. The best use of chemotherapy is for treatment of small amounts of disease left after surgery and radiation.

Multimodality Therapy Essential for Most Adult Cancers. Multimodality therapy, chemotherapy in combination with surgery and radiation, is important for treatment of adult cancer. It allows more cancer cells to be killed, and helps to prevent the development of resistance to chemotherapy or radiation. For instance, surgery is combined with chemotherapy for treating breast and colorectal carcinoma, osteosarcoma, and some types of soft tissue sarcoma; radiation with chemotherapy for Ewing sarcoma, and Hodgkin and certain non-Hodgkin lymphoma;

and radiation with surgery and chemotherapy for head-and-neck, anorectal, breast, cervix, small cell and non–small cell lung carcinoma, and Ewing sarcoma.

Avoiding Radiation Less of an Issue in Adults. There is less constraint for using radiation for treatment of adults with cancer because it does not cause the severe cosmetic, growth, and functional problems seen in growing children. Nor does radiation to a mature brain cause the severe intellectual and learning problems that complicate radiation to a developing brain. Preoperative radiation may be used at diagnosis to make inoperable tumors removable. Very aggressive surgery is sometimes avoided because patients can be treated with postoperative radiation. Postoperative radiation is also given frequently for possible microscopic disease.

Some Adult Cancers Totally Resistant to Chemotherapy. Chemotherapy is generally withheld in those cancers known to be unresponsive, such as melanoma and pancreatic, biliary tract, renal cell, thyroid, prostate, and hepatocellular carcinoma, so as to avoid toxicity without benefit.

Some Adult Cancers Resistant to Both Chemotherapy and Radiation. Malignant central nervous system tumors, such glioblastoma multiforme, malignant astrocytoma, oligodendroglioma, and ependymoma, generally do not respond to chemotherapy or radiation. Also, total resection is usually impossible because of extensive infiltration into the surrounding brain and vital structures, such as the brain stem that controls cardiovascular and respiratory functions and the nerves supplying the face and body. Chemotherapy is generally withheld; radiation may prolong life, although tumor control is seldom long-lasting.

Palliative Chemotherapy and Radiation. Chemotherapy often provides temporary control of pain and symptoms from cancers that cannot be removed surgically or destroyed by radiation. They include bladder, stomach, colorectal, cervix, uterine, pancreatic, adrenocortical, head-and-neck, and breast carcinoma, chronic myelogenous leukemia, hairy cell leukemia, chronic lymphocytic leukemia, low-grade lymphoma, and multiple myeloma. For some of these cancers, radiation may also provide useful palliation.

Pediatric-Type Cancers in Adults Respond Poorly to Treatment. Pediatric-type embryonal, hematologic, and lymphatic malignancies are rare in adults but when they occur act differently from their childhood counterparts. They tend to arise from more mature precursor cells, have poorer biology from acquiring more unfavorable mutations, respond poorly to treatment, and are less curable than the same disease in children. For instance, unlike children, adults usually develop acute myelogenous leukemia, chronic myelogenous leukemia, and chronic lymphocytic leukemia rather than acute lymphoblastic leukemia. If adults develop acute lymphoblastic leukemia, their response to chemotherapy is poorer than in children. Adults also tend to develop chronic types of lymphoma that respond poorly to chemotherapy. If soft tissue sarcoma occurs in adults, it commonly arises from mature tissues, such as from fat (liposarcoma), muscle (leiomyosarcoma), nerve (neurogenic sarcoma), blood vessel (angiosarcoma), and supporting tissues (malignant fibrous histiocytoma, synovial sarcoma, fibrosarcoma, epithelioid sarcoma, malignant soft part sarcoma), and does not respond to chemotherapy or radiation. Adults with rhabdomyosarcoma generally develop the poor-prognosis pleomorphic and alveolar forms that are resistant to chemotherapy and radiation, rather than the embryonal form of childhood that responds to chemotherapy. Bone sarcoma in adults commonly arises from cartilage (chondrosarcoma) and has a more indolent course and poorer response to chemotherapy than the osteosarcoma and Ewing sarcoma of childhood.

Unfavorable Biology of Adult Cancers. As stated, initiation of a cancer in an adult often depends on the accumulation of seven or more mutations in the same cell. In general, most adult cancers acquire more unfavorable mutations of onco-genes and tumor suppressor genes than do childhood cancers. Such mutations result in a poor biology, which means an increased aggressiveness of the cancer, causing the disease to progress early, recur and spread, and respond poorly to chemotherapy and radiation.

Principles of Treatment of Adult Cancers

General Principles. Most adults with cancer are treated on clinical trials or with standard regimens if no clinical trial is open, under the auspices of one of the cooperative groups listed in the appendix. It has been shown that treatment in cancer centers participating in cooperative group clinical trials results in the highest cure rates for each type of cancer. The mandate of cooperative groups is to improve results and reduce treatment side effects and death. It has also been shown that multimodality therapy produces the best results and that combination chemotherapy works better than single-agent chemotherapy. Unlike for children, drug doses in adults are aimed at causing less severe pancytopenia, since adults do not tolerate chemotherapy as well as children. Bone marrow recovery is slower in adults than in children, so chemotherapy cycles are usually repeated every four weeks. Therefore, treatment is generally less intense for adults than for children. Drug doses are also calculated to avoid severe and irreversible damage to the kidneys, liver, brain, nerves, hearing, and bowel lining. As with children, cure is unlikely after relapse from first-line therapy, but second- or third-line therapy may prolong life span.

Curability of the Common Adult Cancers. Skin cancer is by far the most common malignancy, with an incidence that has risen sharply since suntanning became fashionable. About one in five Americans develops skin cancer during their lifetime. About one million new cases of skin cancer occur every year in the United States and 47,000 new cases of melanoma. In addition, another 1.2 million new cases of other cancers are diagnosed each year in the United States. This means that about 500 out of 100,000 adults develop cancer every year, according to SEERS (Surveillance, Epidemiology, and End Results program) statistics. Table 8.1 summarizes the twenty-four most common cancers by annual incidence, order of frequency, primary and relapse therapy, and treatment results expressed as overall five-year relative survival rates (the proportions of patients alive five years after diagnosis, relative to the proportions of the general population expected to live that long). Separate numbers for individuals that are disease-free are not available, but cure rates are probably very close to five-year relative survival rates. The five-year relative survival rates are also quoted separately for localized, regional, and metastatic disease, because localized disease (Stage I) and regional disease (Stage II) are mostly cured, whereas, despite intensive therapy, extensive disease (Stage III) and metastatic disease (Stage IV) are not. Malignancies curable in the early stages include leukemia (acute lymphoblastic and myelogenous, chronic myelogenous), lymphoma (Hodgkin and non-Hodgkin), multiple myeloma, germ cell tumors, soft tissue sarcoma (embryonal rhabdomyosarcoma), bone sarcoma (osteosarcoma, Ewing sarcoma), and carcinoma (prostate, breast, lung, colon, bladder, uterus, ovary, skin, anorectal, oropharyngeal, kidney, cervix, stomach, liver, biliary tract, and esophagus).

Primary and Second-Line Chemotherapy. A full description of the chemotherapy protocols is beyond the scope of this book, but table 8.2 provides a brief summary of those

Table 8.1 Summary of the Twenty-four Most Common Adult Cancers and Treatment Outcomes

Rank	Subtypes	Primary Therapies	Relapse Therapies	Five-year Relative Survival Rates
1	**Nonmelanoma skin cancer (282.3/100,000 persons/year)**			
	(1) basal cell, squamous cell carcinoma	(1) surgery	(1) surgery	90% overall
	(2) precancerous lesions	(2) electrodesiccation	(2) preventive therapy	metastatic 5%
	(3) rare Merkel cell tumor, atypical fibroxanthoma, microcystic adnexal or sebaceous carcinoma, Kaposi sarcoma, malignant fibrous histiocytoma, dermatofibrosarcoma protuberans	(3) liquid nitrogen cryosurgery	(3) molecular therapy	regional 80%
		(4) high-energy pulsed-CO_2 laser therapy		localized 100%
		(5) radiation		
2	**Prostate carcinoma (136/100,000 persons/year)**			
	(1) adenocarcinoma	(1) surgery	(1) surgery	90% overall
	(2) epithelial, nonepithelial tumors	(2) cryosurgery	(2) radiation	metastatic 5%
		(3) radiation	(3) chemotherapy	regional 96%
		(4) surgical or chemical castration	(4) preventive therapy	localized 100%
		(5) [89]strontium or [153]samarium	(5) biologic therapy	

(Continued)

Table 8.1 (Continued)

Rank	Subtypes	Primary Therapies	Relapse Therapies	Five-year Relative Survival Rates
		for bone metastasis	(6) molecular therapy (7) bisphosphonate for osteoporosis	
3	**Breast carcinoma (111/100,000 persons/year)** (1) intraductal *in situ*, invasive intraductal, comedo, medullary-lymphocytic, inflammatory, mucinous, papillary, scirrhous, tubular carcinoma (2) lobular *in situ*, invasive *in situ*, invasive carcinoma (3) Paget disease, Paget with intraductal carcinoma of nipple	(1) surgery (2) radiation (3) surgical or radiation ovarian ablation (4) chemotherapy (5) hormonal therapy for estrogen receptor-negative	(1) surgery (2) radiation (3) chemotherapy (4) auto/alloBMT (5) biologic therapy: anti-Her2/neu antibody (trastuzumab) (6) preventive therapy (7) molecular therapy	85% overall metastatic 5% regional 77% localized 97%
4	**Lung carcinoma (54.2/100,000 persons/year)** Non–small cell lung (26.5/100,000 persons/year): squamous, adenocarcinoma, large cell, adenosquamous,	(1) surgery (2) radiation (3) chemotherapy (4) biologic therapy	(1) surgery (2) radiation (3) chemotherapy (4) biologic therapy	14% overall metastatic 0% regional 20% localized 50%

mixed carcinoma

Small cell lung (27.7/100,000 persons/year): pure small cell, mixed small and large cell, combined small cell carcinoma

(1) surgery
(2) radiation
(3) chemotherapy

(5) preventive therapy
(1) surgery
(2) radiation
(3) chemotherapy
(4) auto/alloBMT
(5) immunotherapy
(6) preventive therapy

5% overall
metastatic 0%
regional 5%
localized 30%

5 **Colon cancer (30.3/100,000 persons/year)**
mucinous, signet ring, adenosquamous, squamous, small cell, medullary carcinoma, choriocarcinoma

(1) surgery
(2) radiation
(3) chemotherapy
(4) transarterial chemotherapy for liver metastasis

(1) surgery
(2) radiation
(3) chemotherapy
(4) immunotherapy
(5) biologic therapy
(6) preventive therapy

62% overall
metastatic 1%
regional 68%
localized 92%

6 **Uterine cancer (21.1/100,000 persons/year)**
(1) papillary endometrioid, papillary serous, endometrioid, clear cell, mucinous carcinoma
(2) endometrial stromal sarcoma, leiomyosarcoma
(3) mixed Müllerian tumor, adenosarcoma

(1) surgery
(2) radiation
(3) chemotherapy
(4) hormonal therapy

(1) surgery
(2) radiation
(3) chemotherapy
(4) preventive therapy

84% overall
metastatic 0%
regional 66%
localized 95%

(*Continued*)

Table 8.1 (*Continued*)

Rank	Subtypes	Primary Therapies	Relapse Therapies	Five-year Relative Survival Rates
	(4) small cell neuroendocrine, squamous cell carcinoma, melanoma, adenocarcinoma, sarcoma of vagina (5) hydatidiform mole, invasive mole, choriocarcinoma, placental trophoblastic disease			
7	**Lymphoma (17.7/100,000 persons/year)** Non-Hodgkin (15.5/100,000 persons/year): (1) B cells: lymphocytic, lymphoplasmacytic, hairy cell, follicular, mantle cell, plasmacytoma, marginal zone B-cell, Burkitt, diffuse large cell (2) T cells: human T-cell lymphotrophic virus type I, natural killer T-cell, anaplastic	(1) chemotherapy (2) CNS prophylaxis: intrathecal chemotherapy (3) radiation (4) mycosis fungoides: topical chemotherapy	(1) chemotherapy (2) auto/alloBMT (3) palliative radiation	51% overall

	Histology/Type	Treatment		5-Year Survival
	large T/null-cell, angioim-munoblastic, mycosis fungoides/cutaneous T-cell lymphoma/Sézary syndrome Hodgkin (2.1/100,000 persons/year): (1) lymphocyte-predominant or rich (2) nodular sclerosis (3) mixed cellularity (4) lymphocyte-depleted (5) unclassifiable	(1) chemotherapy (2) radiation (local, regional, extended-field, or total-nodal)	(1) chemotherapy (2) auto/alloBMT (3) palliative radiation	80% overall metastatic 50% regional 70% localized 90%
8	**Bladder cancer (16.2/100,000 persons/year)** (1) transitional cell, squamous cell, small cell, mixed carcinoma, adenocarcinoma (2) lymphoma, melanoma	(1) surgery (2) radiation (3) laser therapy (4) intrabladder chemotherapy (5) chemotherapy	(1) surgery (2) laser therapy (3) palliative radiation (4) chemotherapy (5) biologic therapy (6) preventive therapy	81% overall metastatic 0% regional 51% localized 93%
9	**Ovarian cancer (14.1/100,000 persons/year)** (1) serous, mucinous, endometrioid carcinoma	(1) surgery (2) radiation	(1) palliative surgery (2) chemotherapy	40% overall metastatic 0%

(Continued)

Table 8.1 (*Continued*)

Rank	Subtypes	Primary Therapies	Relapse Therapies	Five-year Relative Survival Rates
	(2) gonadoblastoma, androblastoma, granulosa-stromal cell, germ cell, lipid cell tumor	(3) chemotherapy (4) intraperitoneal drugs, ^{32}chromic phosphate radioisotope	(3) palliative radiation (4) auto/alloBMT (5) biologic therapy (6) molecular therapy	regional 78% localized 95%
10	**Malignant melanoma (13.8/100,000 persons/year)** lentigo maligna, nodular, subungual, superficial spreading, acral lentiginous, desmoplastic melanoma	(1) surgery (2) CO_2 laser ablation (3) radiation (4) chemotherapy	(1) surgery (2) chemotherapy (3) immunotherapy (4) isolated limb-perfusion and intra-arterial chemotherapy	88% overall metastatic 0% regional 58% localized 95%
11	**Anorectal cancer (12.5/100,000 persons/year)** (1) rectal mucinous, signet ring, squamous, adenosquamous, small cell, medullary carcinoma (2) anal adenocarcinoma, squamous, papillary villous,	(1) surgery (2) radiation (3) chemotherapy	(1) surgery (2) chemotherapy (3) palliative radiation (4) preventive therapy	60% overall metastatic 0% regional 57% localized 85%

transitional carcinoma, melanoma

12 Oropharyngeal cancer (10/100,000 persons/year)

(1) squamous cell, minor salivary gland carcinoma

(2) melanoma, plasmacytoma, sarcoma

(1) surgery
(2) radiation
(3) chemotherapy
(4) remove premalignant dysplasia, hyperplasia, leukoplakia, erythroplakia

(1) surgery
(2) biologic therapy
(3) palliative radiation
(4) molecular therapy
(5) preventive therapy

53% overall
metastatic 0%
regional 43%
localized 81%

13 Leukemia (9.7/100,000 persons/year)

Acute lymphoblastic leukemia (1.3/100,000 persons/year):

(1) Burkitt, precursor, and common B-cell
(2) lymphoblastic T-cell
(3) biphenotypic: lymphoblastic-myelogenous

(1) chemotherapy
(2) CNS prophylaxis: intrathecal chemotherapy
(3) alloBMT

(1) chemotherapy
(2) palliative radiation
(3) 2nd alloBMT
(4) immunotherapy

43% overall

Other leukemia (2.1/100,000 persons/year):

(1) acute undifferentiated
(2) B-cell, hairy cell
(3) prolymphocytic, granular lymphocytic T-cell, natural

(1) chemotherapy
(2) CNS prophylaxis: intrathecal chemotherapy
(3) alloBMT

(1) chemotherapy
(2) palliative radiation
(3) 2nd alloBMT
(4) immunotherapy

20% overall

(*Continued*)

Table 8.1 (Continued)

Rank	Subtypes	Primary Therapies	Relapse Therapies	Five-year Relative Survival Rates
	killer cell, human T-cell lymphotrophic virus type I			
	Acute myelogenous leukemia (2.5/100,000 persons/year): M0, undifferentiated; M1, poorly differentiated; M2, M3, differentiated; M4, myelomonoblastic; M5, monoblastic; M6, erythroblastic; M7, megakaryoblastic	(1) chemotherapy (2) CNS prophylaxis: intrathecal chemotherapy (3) auto/alloBMT	(1) chemotherapy (2) 2nd alloBMT	30% overall
	Chronic myelogenous leukemia (1.5/100,000 persons/year)	(1) chemotherapy (2) alloBMT	(1) chemotherapy (2) 2nd alloBMT (3) immunotherapy (4) biologic therapy (5) molecular therapy	60% overall
	Chronic lymphocytic leukemia (2.3/100,000 persons/year): (1) chronic lymphocytic B-cell (2) prolymphocytic B-cell	(1) supportive therapy (2) chemotherapy (3) splenectomy or splenic radiation	(1) chemotherapy (2) immunotherapy (3) alloBMT (4) molecular therapy	0% overall, disease stable for years, dying of unrelated causes

14	**Renal carcinoma (9.4/100,000 persons/year)**		
	(1) clear cell, papillary, collecting duct carcinoma, oncocytoma, chromophobe, sarcomatoid tumor of kidney	(1) surgery	(1) surgery	60% overall
		(2) radiation	(2) chemotherapy	metastatic 5%
		(3) chemotherapy	(3) palliative radiation	regional 62%
		(4) biologic therapy	(4) biologic therapy	localized 88%
	(2) squamous cell, transitional cell, mixed transitional cell, undifferentiated carcinoma, adenocarcinoma, leiomyosarcoma of renal pelvis and ureter	(5) alloBMT	(5) molecular therapy	
15	**Pancreatic cancer (8.6/100,000 persons/year)**		
	(1) exocrine ductal, mucinous, acinar, unclassified large cell, small cell carcinoma, cystadenocarcinoma, pancreatoblastoma	(1) surgery	(1) surgery	4% overall
		(2) radiation	(2) chemotherapy	metastatic 0%
		(3) radiation with radiosensitizing chemotherapy: paclitaxel, gemcitabine	(3) intra-arterial chemotherapy for local recurrence and liver metastases	regional 6%
	(2) endocrine gastrinoma, insulinoma, PPoma (pancreatic polypeptide), VIPoma (vasoactive intestinal peptide), glucagonoma, GRFoma (growth hormone-releasing factor),	(4) chemotherapy	(4) palliative radiation	localized 17%
		(5) hormone therapy		
		(6) biologic therapy		

(Continued)

Table 8.1 (*Continued*)

Rank	Subtypes	Primary Therapies	Relapse Therapies	Five-year Relative Survival Rates
	somatostatinoma, ACTHoma (adrenocorticotropic hormone) (3) mucinous cystadenoma, intraductal papillary mucinous, papillary cystic tumor			
16	**Cervix cancer (7.7/100,000 persons/year)**			
	(1) *in situ*, microinvasive, invasive adenocarcinoma	(1) surgery (2) radiation	(1) surgery (2) chemotherapy	71% overall metastatic 0%
	(2) preinvasive, invasive squamous cell carcinoma	(3) chemotherapy (4) intra-arterial chemotherapy	(3) palliative radiation (4) preventive therapy	regional 49% localized 91%
	(3) potentially invasive intraepithelial lesion			
17	**Stomach cancer (6.6/100,000 persons/year)**			
	(1) adenocarcinoma	(1) surgery	(1) surgery	21% overall
	(2) squamous cell carcinoma	(2) radiation	(2) chemotherapy	metastatic 0%
	(3) adenoacanthoma, carcinoid, leiomyosarcoma	(3) chemotherapy (4) hyperthermic peritoneal chemotherapy (5) immunotherapy	(3) palliative radiation (4) preventive therapy	regional 21% localized 62%

18 **Brain and spinal cord tumors (5.8/100,000 persons/year)**

(1) malignant astrocytoma, glioblastoma multiforme (GBM), oligodendroglioma, oligoastrocytoma, brain stem glioma
(2) ependymoma, ependymoblastoma
(3) medulloblastoma
(4) choroid plexus carcinoma, meningioma, primitive germ cell, malignant nerve sheath, chordoma
(5) astrocytoma, ependymoma, schwannoma, meningioma, chordoma, sarcoma, carcinoma, lymphoma of spine cord

(1) surgery
(2) ventriculo peritoneal shunt for increased intracranial pressure
(3) radiation
(4) chemotherapy
(5) gamma knife radiosurgery
(6) intra-arterial chemotherapy
(7) intraventricular chemotherapy

(1) surgery
(2) chemotherapy
(3) palliative radiation
(4) biologic therapy
(5) auto/alloBMT for medulloblastoma

31% overall
GMB 0%

19 **Liver and biliary tract cancer (4.2/100,000 persons/year)**

(1) well-differentiated, moderately differentiated, poorly differentiated, clear cell, fibrolamellar hepatocellular carcinoma

(1) surgery
(2) chemotherapy
(3) liver transplant
(4) radiation
(5) intra-arterial chemotherapy

(1) surgery
(2) chemotherapy
(3) palliative radiation
(4) biologic therapy
(5) auto/alloBMT for

5% overall
metastatic 0%
regional 5%
localized 16%

(Continued)

Table 8.1. (*Continued*)

Rank	Subtypes	Primary Therapies	Relapse Therapies	Five-year Relative Survival Rates
	(2) carcinoid, cholangiocarcinoma of biliary tract	(6) arterial embolization (drugs, ^{90}yttrium-microspheres) (7) cryosurgery, microwave ablation, percutaneous ethanol or acetic acid injection (8) hormonal therapy (9) immunotherapy	medulloblastoma	
20	Multiple myeloma (4.2/100,000 persons/year) plasmacytoma, multiple myeloma, monoclonal gammopathy, Waldenström macroglobulinemia	(1) chemotherapy (2) radiation (3) alloBMT	(1) chemotherapy (2) palliative radiation (3) molecular therapy	29% overall
21	Esophageal cancer (4/100,000 persons/year) (1) squamous cell, cystic, mucoepidermoid, small cell, adenoid, sarcomatous squamous cell carcinoma, adenocarcinoma (2) leiomyosarcoma, lymphoma, melanoma	(1) surgery (2) radiation (3) chemotherapy (4) biologic therapy	(1) surgery (2) chemotherapy (3) palliative radiation (4) molecular therapy (5) preventive therapy	11% overall metastatic 0% regional 10% localized 24%

22	Soft tissue sarcoma (2.2/100,000 persons/year)		
	(1) embryonal, undifferentiated, alveolar, mixed, pleomorphic rhabdomyosarcoma	(1) chemotherapy	
		(2) surgery	
		(3) radiation	
	(2) angiosarcoma, malignant fibrous histiocytoma, liposarcoma, fibrosarcoma, leiomyosarcoma, synovial, neurogenic, and malignant soft part sarcoma, neurofibrosarcoma, lymphangiosarcoma	(4) auto/alloBMT for metastatic disease	(1) chemotherapy — 50% overall
			(2) surgery — metastatic 5%
			(3) palliative radiation — regional 35%
			(4) auto/alloBMT — localized 70%
			(5) biologic therapy
			(6) immunotherapy
23	Testicular cancer (1.7/100,000 persons/year)		
	(1) seminoma, embryonal carcinoma, teratoma, yolk sac tumor, choriocarcinoma	(1) chemotherapy	
		(2) surgery	
		(3) radiation	
	(2) Leydig cell, Sertoli cell, granulosa cell tumor	(4) hormonal therapy	(1) chemotherapy — 70% overall
	(3) gonadoblastoma		(2) surgery — metastatic 50%
	(4) mesothelioma, adenocarcinoma of rete testis		(3) palliative radiation — regional 80%
	(5) carcinoid, sarcoma, lymphoma		(4) auto/alloBMT — localized 90%

(Continued)

Table 8.1 (*Continued*)

Rank	Subtypes	Primary Therapies	Relapse Therapies	Five-year Relative Survival Rates
24	**Bone sarcoma (0.73/100,000 persons/year)**			
	(1) osteosarcoma, chondrosarcoma	(1) chemotherapy	(1) chemotherapy	50% overall
	(2) Ewing sarcoma, primitive peripheral neuroectodermal tumor (PNET)	(2) surgery	(2) surgery	metastatic 5%
	(3) malignant giant cell tumor, adamantinoma, hemangioendothelioma, hemangiopericytoma	(3) radiation	(3) palliative radiation	regional 50%
		(4) auto/alloBMT for metastatic Ewing sarcoma	(4) auto/alloBMT for Ewing sarcoma and PNET	localized 70%

Abbreviations: autoBMT is autologous bone marrow/stem cell transplant; alloBMT is allogeneic bone marrow/stem cell transplant. Result of treatment is measured as the estimated five-year relative survival rate, which means the proportion of patients alive five years from diagnosis (in remission or relapsed), compared to the proportion in the general population expected to live that long. In general, localized disease has favorable biology and is good-risk, metastatic disease has unfavorable biology and is poor-risk disease, and regional disease is intermediate-risk with favorable or unfavorable biology.

Table 8.2 Primary and Second-line Chemotherapy for Twenty-Four Adult Cancers

Incidence Rank	Primary Chemotherapy and Other Therapy for Newly Diagnosed Cancers	Second-line Chemotherapy and Other Therapy for Relapsed Cancers	Death Rank	Death Rates
1	**Nonmelanoma skin cancer** no available chemotherapy	(1) molecular therapy (2) preventive therapy: use sunscreens, vitamin A derivatives (retinoids, carotenoids), and selenium, low-calorie/high-antioxidant diet	24	annual death rate not available
2	**Prostate cancer** (1) chemotherapy: mitoxantrone-prednisone (2) androgen deprivation: gonadotrophin-releasing hormone analogues, estrogens, steroids, antiandrogens, adrenal androgen inhibitors, peripheral testosterone blockade (3) bone metastasis: [89]strontium or [153]samarium radioisotopes	(1) chemotherapy: mitoxantrone, estramustine, vinblastine, docetaxel, paclitaxel, doxorubicin, cyclophosphamide, vinorelbine, carboplatin, etoposide, 5-fluorouracil, mitomycin C (2) molecular therapy: growth factors, their receptors, and their signaling pathways, differentiation therapy, antiangiogenic therapy, antimetastatic therapy, immunotherapy (3) preventive therapy: low-fat plant and soy-based diet with green tea	3	24.1/100,000 persons/year

(Continued)

Table 8.2 (*Continued*)

Incidence Rank	Primary Chemotherapy and Other Therapy for Newly Diagnosed Cancers	Second-line Chemotherapy and Other Therapy for Relapsed Cancers	Death Rank	Death Rates
	(4) osteoporosis: bisphosphonates	and tomato (the carotenoid lycopene), avoid inactivity, use vitamins E and D and selenium		
3	**Breast cancer** (1) chemotherapy: cyclophosphamide, 5-fluorouracil, methotrexate (CMF); cyclophosphamide, doxorubicin, 5-fluorouracil (CAF) (2) hormonal therapy: antiestrogens (tamoxifen), block ovaries with luteinizing hormone-releasing hormone-like drugs, aromatase inhibitors, progestins, androgens, high-dose estrogens (3) bone metastasis and osteoporosis: bisphosphonates	(1) chemotherapy: docetaxel, mitoxantrone, melphalan, thiotepa, vinblastine, vinorelbine, epirubicin, capecitabine, gemcitabine, 5-fluorouracil-leucovorin (2) biologic therapy: Her2/neu antibody trastuzumab (Herceptin), VEGF angiogenic factor antibody bevacizumab (Avastin) with chemotherapy, immunotherapy (3) molecular therapy: growth factors, their receptors, and their signaling pathways, differentiation therapy, antiangiogenic therapy, antimetastatic therapy	2	24.3/100,000 persons/year

(4) preventive therapy: avoid high estrogen/progestin, avoid inactivity, low-fat/high-fiber diet, use vitamin A derivatives and nonsteroidal anti-inflammatory drugs (aspirin, celecoxib[†])

Lung cancer

4 Non–small cell lung cancer (NSCLC) chemotherapy: cyclophosphamide, doxorubicin, cisplatin (CAP); cisplatin, 5-fluorouracil, leucovorin (PFL); ifosfamide, cisplatin, etoposide (ICE)

(1) chemotherapy: paclitaxel, docetaxol, vinorelbine, vinblastine, vindesine, mitomycin C, gemcitabine, irinotecan, topotecan, tirapazamine

(2) biologic therapy: epidermal growth factor receptor (EGFR) antibodies cetuximab and panitumumab, VEGF angiogenic factor antibody bevacizumab (Avastin) with chemotherapy, *Bacille Calmette-Guérin* (BCG)-levamisole, interferons, interleukins

(3) molecular therapy: epidermal growth factor receptor (EGFR) inhibitors gefitnib (Iressa) and erlotinib (Tarceva)

1

48.8/100,000 persons/year

(*Continued*)

Table 8.2 (*Continued*)

Incidence Rank	Primary Chemotherapy and Other Therapy for Newly Diagnosed Cancers	Second-line Chemotherapy and Other Therapy for Relapsed Cancers	Death Rank	Death Rates
		(4) preventive therapy: use vitamins C, E, and A derivatives and selenium; avoid tobacco, asbestos, and chemical carcinogens		
	Small cell lung cancer (SCLC) chemotherapy: cyclophosphamide, doxorubicin, etoposide (CDE); cyclophosphamide, doxorubicin, vincristine, etoposide (CAVE): ifosfamide, carboplatin, etoposide (ICE)	(1) chemotherapy: vincristine, ifosfamide, cisplatin, etoposide, carboplatin, paclitaxel (2) biologic therapy: SCLC antibodies, BCG-levamisole, interferons, interleukins, anticoagulants (Coumadin, heparin) (3) preventive therapy: as for NSCLC		
5	Colon cancer (1) chemotherapy: 5-fluorouracil-leucovorin with other agents (irinotecan, semustine, BCG, vincristine, trimetrexate, methotrexate, uracil, tegafur) (2) intra-arterial therapy for liver metastasis: mitomycin C, oxaliplatin,	(1) chemotherapy: irinotecan, oxaliplatin, capecitabine, eniluracil (2) biologic therapy: tumor antigen antibody (17–1A), thymidine synthetase inhibition (raltitrexed, 5-fluorouracil-leucovorin), EGFR antibodies cetuximab and	4	14.4/100,000 persons/year

#	Treatment		Number	Incidence
	irinotecan, raltitrexed, floxuridine (3) immunotherapy: BCG-levamisole, tumor-cell vaccines, interferon-α_{2a}	panitumumab, VEGF angiogenic factor antibody bevacizumab (Avastin) with chemotherapy (3) preventive therapy: high-fiber/low-alcohol/calcium-supplemented diet, avoid tobacco, use vitamins C, E, and A derivatives, selenium, and nonsteriodal anti-inflammatory drugs (aspirin, celecoxib[†])		
6	**Uterine cancer** chemotherapy: cyclophosphamide, doxorubicin, 5-fluorouracil (CAF); Taxol, doxorubicin, cisplatin (TAP); melphalan, 5-fluorouracil (MEL)	(1) chemotherapy: epirubicin, ifosfamide, etoposide, paclitaxel, carboplatin (2) hormonal therapy: antiestrogens, high-dose progestrogen, luteinizing hormone-releasing hormone-like drugs, aromatase inhibitor	14	3.3/100,000 persons/year
7	**Lymphoma** Non-Hodgkin lymphoma: (1) chemotherapy: cyclophosphamide, doxorubicin, vincristine, prednisone (CHOP); bleomycin, doxorubicin, cyclophosphamide, vincristine,	(1) chemotherapy: dexamethasone, cytarabine, cisplatin, chlorambucil, cyclophosphamide, fludarabine, cladribine, mitoxantrone, epirubicin, idarubicin, teniposide, etoposide,	7	6.9/100,000 persons/year

(Continued)

Table 8.2 (*Continued*)

Incidence Rank	Primary Chemotherapy and Other Therapy for Newly Diagnosed Cancers	Second-line Chemotherapy and Other Therapy for Relapsed Cancers	Death Rank	Death Rates
	prednisone (BACOP); prednisone, methotrexate, leucovorin, dcxorubicin, cyclophosphamide, etoposide, cytarabine, bleomycin, vincristine (ProMACE-CytaBOM) (2) CNS prophylaxis: cytarabine, methotrexate, hydrocortisone (3) topical therapy for mycosis fungoides: carmustine, Mustargen, photochemotherapy Hodgkin lymphoma: chemotherapy: Mustargen, vincristine, procarbazine, prednisone (MOPP); cyclophosphamide, vincristine, procarbazine, prednisone (COPP); doxorubicin, bleomycin, vinblastine, dacarbazine (ABVD); MOPP/ABV hybrid (no dacarbazine); bleomycin, etoposide, doxorubicin, cyclophosphamide, vincristine, procarbazine, prednisone (BEACOPP)	vinblastine, vindesine, irinotecan, topotecan, camptothecin, ifosfamide, carboplatin (2) mycosis fungoides: retinoids, anti-CD4 or anti-CD5 antibodies, fusion toxins, 2'-deoxycoformycin (3) biologic therapy: anti-CD20 antibody (rituximab), interferon-α, BCL-2 antisense antibody, tumor vaccines (1) chemotherapy: daunorubicin, mitoxantrone, epirubicin, idarubicin, ifosfamide, etoposide, carboplatin, vindesine, camptothecin, irinotecan, topotecan, vinorelbine, gemcitabine (2) biologic therapy: CD16/CD30 antibodies, CD25 or CD30 immunotoxin, ^{99m}Tc anti-CD30 radioimmunoconjugate,		

interleukin-2, interferon-α, BCG, lymphokine-activated killer cells (LAK cell)

(3) gene therapy: Epstein-Barr virus (EBV)/lymphocytes containing EBV-specific cytotoxin

8   **Bladder cancer**

(1) chemotherapy: cisplatin, vinblastine, methotrexate (CMV); methotrexate, vinblastine, doxorubicin, cisplatin (M-VAC); ifosfamide, paclitaxel, cisplatin (ITP)

(2) intrabladder therapy: thiotepa, doxorubicin, mitomycin C, BCG, interleukins, interferons

(1) chemotherapy: paclitaxel, cisplatin, methotrexate, vinblastine

(2) biologic therapy: interferon-α/cisplatin, 5-fluorouracil, immunotherapy, cytokine therapy

(3) preventive therapy: diet low in fried meat and fat, use pyridoxine, vitamins C, E, and A derivatives, and zinc, avoid tobacco, phenacetin, and chemical carcinogens

15   3.2/100,000 persons/year

9   **Ovarian cancer**

(1) chemotherapy: cyclophosphamide, doxorubicin, cisplatin (CAP); cyclophosphamide, hexamethylmelamine, doxorubicin, carboplatin (CHAP)

(1) chemotherapy: paclitaxel, carboplatin, gemcitabine, topotecan, etoposide, gemcitabine, liposomal doxorubicin, vinorelbine, hexamethylmelamine, ifosfamide

6   7.4/100,000 persons/year

(Continued)

Table 8.2 (*Continued*)

Incidence Rank	Primary Chemotherapy and Other Therapy for Newly Diagnosed Cancers	Second-line Chemotherapy and Other Therapy for Relapsed Cancers	Death Rank	Death Rates
	(2) intraperitoneal therapy: hyperthermic drugs (carboplatin, paclitaxel) or radioisotopes (^{32}chromic phosphate) (3) hormonal therapy: antiestrogens (tamoxifen), progestins (4) immunotherapy: immunostimulants, IL-2/LAK cells, radioimmunoconjugates	(2) multidrug resistance reversal therapy for P-glycoprotein at present; future possibilities: blocking MRP, LRP, modulating topoisomerase II and glutathione-S-transferase enzyme activity, targeting overactive DNA repair enzymes		
10	Malignant melanoma (1) chemotherapy: cisplatin, vinblastine, dacarbazine (CVD); cisplatin, vinblastine, dacarbazine, tamoxifen (CVDT) (2) intra-arterial chemotherapy: cisplatin (3) hyperthermic limb perfusion: thiotepa, melphalan, cisplatin, dactinomycin, dacarbazine, mitoxantrone, etoposide, IL-2, interferon-γ, tumor necrosis factor (TNF-α), LAK cells	(1) chemotherapy: Taxol, dibromodulcitol, carmustine, lomustine, semustine, fotemustine, vincristine, vindesine, carboplatin, temozolomide, cyclophosphamide, bleomycin (2) immunotherapy: stimulate immunity (BCG-levamisole, *Corynebacterium parvum*), interferons, vaccines (ganglioside	20	2.3/100,000 persons/year

(4) chemotherapy-biologic therapy: CVD
    with IL-2 or interferon
(5) hormonal therapy: antiestrogen
    (tamoxifen)

GM2 antibody, tumor cell-derived
and melanoma antigen vaccines),
local BCG, interferon-α injections
to induce immunity

11	**Anorectal cancer** (1) chemotherapy: 5-fluorouracil, leucovorin, levamisole (FLL); semustine, vincristine, 5-fluorouracil (MOF) (2) radiosensitizing therapy: 5-fluorouracil, razoxane, hyperthermia (3) radioprotective therapy: WR-2721, 5-aminosalicylic acid, sucralfate enema, caffeine, elemental diet, sodium pentosanpolysulfate, butyric acid	(1) chemotherapy: raltitrexed, camptothecin, oxaliplatin, tegafur, uracil, high-dose methotrexate-leucovorin, mitomycin C, cisplatin, doxorubicin, cisplatin, carboplatin, bleomycin, vincristine (2) preventive therapy: see colon cancer	19 2.4/100,000 persons/year
12	**Oropharyngeal cancer** (1) chemotherapy: cisplatin/5-fluorouracil/ methotrexate/bleomycin; paclitaxel/ cisplatin/5-fluorouracil/ifosfamide/ gemcitabine (2) chemotherapy-biologic therapy: drugs with IL-2 or interferon	(1) chemotherapy: epirubicin, vincristine, vinblastine, docetaxel, vinorelbine (2) molecular therapy: growth factors, their receptors, and their signaling pathways, *p53* gene	18 2.6/100,000 persons/year

(Continued)

Table 8.2 (*Continued*)

Incidence Rank	Primary Chemotherapy and Other Therapy for Newly Diagnosed Cancers	Second-line Chemotherapy and Other Therapy for Relapsed Cancers	Death Rank	Death Rates
		therapy to restore tumor suppressor activity		
13	**Leukemia**			
	Acute lymphoblastic leukemia:	(1) chemotherapy: doxorubicin, etoposide, teniposide, mitoxantrone, epirubicin, idarubicin, vinblastine, vindesine, irinotecan, topotecan, camptothecin	8	6.3/100,000 persons/year
	(1) *Induction*: prednisone/dexamethasone, vincristine, daunorubicin, asparaginase			
	(2) *Consolidation*: cyclophosphamide, high-dose methotrexate, high-dose cytarabine, doxorubicin, cytarabine, asparaginase	(2) biologic therapy: interferon (hairy cell leukemia), monoclonal antibodies, vaccines		
	(3) *CNS prophylaxis*: cytarabine, methotrexate, hydrocortisone			
	(4) *Maintenance and reinduction*: methotrexate, mercaptopurine, thioguanine, prednisone, vincristine			
	Acute myelogenous leukemia:	(1) chemotherapy: doxorubicin, etoposide, teniposide, mitoxantrone, epirubicin, idarubicin, vinblastine,		
	(1) *Induction*: daunorubicin, cytarabine, cytarabine or high-dose cytarabine			

(2) *Maintenance:* daunorubicin, cytarabine or high-dose cytarabine, thioguanine
(3) *CNS prophylaxis:* intrathecal cytarabine
(4) *Induction and maintenance for M3 acute promyelocytic leukemia:* all-*trans*-retinoic acid (ATRA), idarubicin, cytarabine, mitoxantrone, etoposide

Chronic myelogenous leukemia:
(1) busulfan, hydroxyurea
(2) chemotherapy-biologic therapy: cytarabine with interferon

Chronic lymphocytic leukemia: chemotherapy: chlorambucil, prednisone (CP); cyclophosphamide, doxorubicin, vincristine, prednisone (CHOP); single

vindesine, irinotecan, topotecan, camptothecin
(2) biologic therapy: interferon, IL-2, monoclonal antibodies, vaccines

(1) chemotherapy: daunorubicin, doxorubicin, mitoxantrone, epirubicin, idarubicin, high-dose cytarabine, homoharringtonine
(2) molecular therapy: block ABL kinase with imatinib (Gleevec), dasatinib (Sprycel), and nilotinib (Tasigna), block tyrosine kinase enzyme and G-protein receptor signaling pathways (see chapter 9), *ABL-BCR* antisense oligonucleotides, deoxycytidine inducing DNA demethylation

(1) chemotherapy: fludarabine, cytarabine, chlorambucil, 2-chlorodeoxyadenosine, 2'-deoxycoformycin, cisplatin

(*Continued*)

Table 8.2 (*Continued*)

Incidence Rank	Primary Chemotherapy and Other Therapy for Newly Diagnosed Cancers	Second-line Chemotherapy and Other Therapy for Relapsed Cancers	Death Rank	Death Rates
		agents (fludarabine, chlorambucil, cyclophosphamide, prednisone)	(2) molecular therapy: target signaling pathways, apoptosis-inducing arsenic (3) biologic therapy: interferon, CD52 antibody (Campath-1) and CD20 antibody (rituximab)		
14	**Renal Cancer** (1) chemotherapy: 5-fluorouracil/gemcitabine; single agents (fluoxuridine, 5-fluorouracil, gemcitabine, 6-thioguanine) (2) immunotherapy: vaccines, interferon-α, IL-2, LAK cells, tumor-infiltrating lymphocytes (3) chemotherapy-biologic therapy: interferon-α with fluoxuridine, 5-fluorouracil, or vinblastine	(1) chemotherapy: paclitaxel, docetaxel, homoharringtonine, LY186641, liposomal doxorubicin, edatrexate, temozolomide (2) hormonal therapy: antiestrogen (tamoxifen), progestin, androgens (3) multidrug resistance reversal therapy for P-glycoprotein (4) antiangiogenic therapy: vascular endothelial growth factor (VEGF) antibody, vinblastine with	13	3.5/100,000 persons/year

nonsteroidal anti-inflammatory
drug celecoxib[†]

15

Pancreatic cancer

(1) chemotherapy: 5-fluorouracil,
doxorubicin, mitomycin C (FAM);
streptozocin, mitomycin C,
5-fluorouracil (SMF);
5-fluorouracil-gemcitabine

(2) hormonal therapy: antiestrogen
(tamoxifen), luteinizing hormone-
releasing hormone (LHRH) analogue,
somatostatin analogue octretide bound
to yttrium[90] radioisotope or
methotrexate

5

(1) chemotherapy: paclitaxel,
docetaxel, iproplatin, trimetrexate,
edatrexate, fazarabine, diaziquone,
mitoguazone, amonafide,
topotecan, irinotecan

(2) intra-arterial therapy for pancreas
and liver metastases: cisplatin,
5-fluorouracil, mitoxantrone

(3) molecular therapy: farnesyl
transferase inhibition in *ras*
oncogene signaling pathway by
small molecules, epidermal growth
factor receptor (EGFR) inhibition
by C225 antibody

(4) biologic therapy: epidermal growth
factor receptor (EGFR) antibodies
cetuximab and panitumumab

(5) preventive therapy: avoid smoking,
high intake of alcohol and coffee

8.3/100,000
persons/year

(*Continued*)

Table 8.2 (*Continued*)

Incidence Rank	Primary Chemotherapy and Other Therapy for Newly Diagnosed Cancers	Second-line Chemotherapy and Other Therapy for Relapsed Cancers	Death Rank	Death Rates
16	**Cervix Cancer** (1) chemotherapy: bleomycin, vincristine, cisplatin (BOP); bleomycin, vincristine, mitomycin C, cisplatin (BOMP) (2) intra-arterial chemotherapy: 5-fluorouracil, cisplatin	(1) chemotherapy: ifosfamide, doxorubicin, cyclophosphamide, chlorambucil, melphalan, vindesine, vinorelbine, irinotecan, razoxane, topotecan, paclitaxel, carboplatin, ifosfamide (2) preventive therapy: avoid smoking and prolonged oral contraceptives, treat genital papilloma virus infections, use vitamins C and A derivatives	17	2.7/100,000 persons/year
17	**Stomach Cancer** (1) chemotherapy: 5-fluorouracil, doxorubicin, mitomycin C (FAM); mitomycin C, cyclophosphamide, methotrexate, 5-fluorouracil, vincristine (MMC-CMFV)	(1) chemotherapy: 5-fluorouracil-leucovorin, doxorubicin, epirubicin, cisplatin, mitomycin C (2) intraperitoneal therapy: hyperthermic therapy with drugs	10	4.0/100,000 persons/year

(2) hormonal therapy: antiestrogen (tamoxifen)
(3) other therapy: histamine-2 blocker, ranitidine

(mitomycin C, cisplatin)
(3) immunotherapy: bacterial or fungal polysaccharide
(4) preventive therapy: diet high in fiber, fruits, and vegetables and low in salt and nitrate, avoid smoking and chemical carcinogens, use riboflavin, zinc, niacin, vitamins C, E, and A derivatives, molybdenum, selenium, and nonsteroidal anti-inflammatory drugs (aspirin, celecoxib[†])

18 Brain and spinal cord tumor

(1) glioma chemotherapy: procarbazine, lomustine, vincristine (PCV)
(2) medulloblastoma chemotherapy: ifosfamide, carboplatin, etoposide (ICE); Mustargen, vincristine, procarbazine, prednisone (MOPP)
(3) intraventricular drugs: hydrocortisone, methotrexate, cytarabine, thiotepa, topotecan
(4) intracystic drugs: carmustine biodegradable polymers, bleomycin

(1) chemotherapy: prednisone, dexamethasone, paclitaxel, temozolomide, irinotecan, ifosfamide, etoposide, teniposide, vinblastine
(2) intra-arterial chemotherapy: cisplatin, carmustine
(3) biologic therapy: retinoids (all-*trans*-retinoic acid, 13-*cis*-retinoic acid), antiestrogen (tamoxifen), interferon-α and β

9 4.2/100,000 persons/year

(Continued)

Table 8.2 (*Continued*)

Incidence Rank	Primary Chemotherapy and Other Therapy for Newly Diagnosed Cancers	Second-line Chemotherapy and Other Therapy for Relapsed Cancers	Death Rank	Death Rates
19	**Liver and biliary tract** **Hepatocellular carcinoma:** (1) chemotherapy: cisplatin-doxorubicin-5-fluorouracil-interferon, doxorubicin-5-fluorouracil-vincristine-cyclophosphamide, 5-fluorouracil-leucovorin-hydroxyurea (2) intra-arterial chemotherapy: 5-fluorouracil-methotrexate-cisplatin-interferon, fluorouridine-doxorubicin-streptozotocin, leucovorin-doxorubicin-cisplatin **Cholangiocarcinoma:** chemotherapy: 5-fluorouracil-leucovorin,	(1) chemotherapy: irinotecan, paclitaxel (2) immunotherapy: interferon-α and β (3) chemotherapy-immunotherapy: interferon, cisplatin, doxorubicin, 5-fluorouracil (4) hormonal therapy: antiandrogens, antiestrogens (tamoxifen also blocks P-glycoprotein multidrug resistance), tamoxifen with etoposide, epirubicin or doxorubicin (5) preventive therapy: avoid chemical carcinogens, fungal alfatoxin, alcohol (1) chemotherapy: paclitaxel, carboplatin, streptozotocin	11	3.6/100,000 persons/year

20	5-fluorouracil-leucovorin-methotrexate-epirubicin, 5-fluorouracil-gemcitabine, doxorubicin-carmustine-tegafur (2) chemotherapy-immunotherapy: 5-fluorouracil, interferon-α_{2b} (3) intra-arterial chemotherapy: mitomycin C, 5-fluorouracil, fluorouridine	

Multiple myeloma

	(1) chemotherapy: vincristine, doxorubicin, high-dose dexamethasone (VAD); cyclophosphamide, vincristine, doxorubicin, high-dose dexamethasone (CVAD); vincristine, melphalan, prednisone (VMP) (2) immunotherapy: interferon-α, tumor cell-specific cytotoxic T cells (3) hormonal therapy: antiestrogen (tamoxifen)	16	3.1/100,000 persons/year
	(1) chemotherapy: high-dose dexamethasone, cyclophosphamide, etoposide, cisplatin (DCEP); high-dose dexamethasone, thalidomide, cisplatin, doxorubicin, cyclophosphamide, etoposide (DTPACE) (2) biologic therapy: arsenic trioxide, CD20 antibody (rituximab), antiangiogenic/anti-TNF-α therapy (thalidomide), osteoporosis/metastasis therapy (bisphosphonate) (3) molecular therapy: TNF-α inhibition, target *ras* activity, reduce telomerase activity, farnesyl transferase and geranyl-geranyl transferase inhibition		

(Continued)

Table 8.2 (*Continued*)

Incidence Rank	Primary Chemotherapy and Other Therapy for Newly Diagnosed Cancers	Second-line Chemotherapy and Other Therapy for Relapsed Cancers	Death Rank	Death Rates
21	**Esophageal cancer** (1) chemotherapy: cisplatin with 5-fluorouracil, bleomycin, vindesine, methotrexate, vinorelbine, etoposide, paclitaxel or irinotecan (2) biologic therapy: 13-*cis*-retinoic acid, interferon-α_{2a} (3) chemotherapy-biologic therapy: 5-fluorouracil-interferon-α_{2c}	(1) chemotherapy: carboplatin, vinblastine, cisplatin, irinotecan, paclitaxel (2) molecular therapy: epidermal growth factor erbB2 receptor inhibition, restoring cell cycle arrest and apoptosis (flavopiridol), *RB1, p16, p53, p107* gene therapy to restore tumor suppressor activity, deoxycytidine inducing DNA demethylation, histone deacetylase inhibitors, telomerase inhibition (3) preventive therapy: lose weight, avoid smoking, excess alcohol, strong tea, and fermented vegetables, use vitamins C, E, and A derivatives, riboflavin, zinc, niacin, molybdenum, and selenium	12	3.6/100,000 persons/year

22	**Soft tissue sarcoma** chemotherapy: cyclophosphamide, doxorubicin, methotrexate (CAM); cyclophosphamide, vincristine, doxorubicin, dacarbazine (CyVADIC); ifosfamide, etoposide (IE)	21	1.1/100,000 persons/year
23	**Testicular cancer** chemotherapy: cisplatin, vinblastine, bleomycin (PVB); cisplatin, vinblastine, bleomycin, dactinomycin, cyclophosphamide (VAB); vinblastine, ifosfamide, cisplatin (VIP)	23	0.2/100,000 persons/year
24	**Bone sarcoma** Osteosarcoma, chondrosarcoma: chemotherapy: doxorubicin-cisplatin; high-dose methotrexate-leucovorin; ifosfamide, etoposide (IE)	22	0.36/100,000 persons/year

chemotherapy: epirubicin, idarubicin, mitoxantrone, teniposide, irinotecan, topotecan, camptothecin, cisplatin, carboplatin, ifosfamide, etoposide

chemotherapy: teniposide, vincristine, cyclophosphamide, ifosfamide, doxorubicin, mitoxantrone, epirubicin, idarubicin, irinotecan, topotecan, camptothecin, paclitaxel, gemcitabine, carboplatin

(1) chemotherapy: bleomycin, cyclophosphamide, dactinomycin (BCD); mitoxantrone, epirubicin, idarubicin, teniposide, irinotecan, topotecan, camptothecin
(2) biologic therapy: lung metastases therapy with muramyltripeptide phosphatidylethanolamine

(Continued)

Table 8.2 (*Continued*)

Incidence Rank	Primary Chemotherapy and Other Therapy for Newly Diagnosed Cancers	Second-line Chemotherapy and Other Therapy for Relapsed Cancers	Death Rank	Death Rates
		(MTP-PE) or granulocyte-macrophage colony-stimulating factor (GM-CSF), interferon, BCG		
	Ewing sarcoma, primitive peripheral neuroectodermal tumor (PNET): chemotherapy: vincristine, doxorubicin, cyclophosphamide (VadriaC); vincristine, dactinomycin, cyclophosphamide (VAC); ifosfamide, etoposide (IE)	chemotherapy: mitoxantrone, epirubicin, idarubicin, teniposide, irinotecan, topotecan, camptothecin, cisplatin, carboplatin		

[†]Nonsteroidal anti-inflammatory drugs celecoxib (Celebrex) and rofecoxib (Vioxx) trials are presently on hold to investigate possible increased heart attack risk.

malignancies in which chemotherapy plays a role. Table 8.2 also illustrates the biologic therapy (immunotherapy and hormonal therapy, see chapter 6) and novel targeted therapies (see chapter 9) used to treat each type of cancer. Radiation therapy has been discussed in chapter 5. With the exception of leukemia, lymphoma, and germ cell tumors, the role of chemotherapy is subsidiary to surgery, radiation, and other therapy. Because numerous protocols exist, only one or two main examples are included shown in bold, with the appropriate treatment phases shown in italics. The death rates are the annual numbers of cancer deaths for every 100,000 patients with that particular cancer. Death rates of the different cancers are also ranked for comparison, to highlight those cancers that are major killers. Second-line therapy may consist of alternative chemotherapy, further surgery, radiation, biological therapy, and molecular targeted therapy. Those patients that respond a second time may receive further high-dose consolidation chemotherapy, with marrow rescue by autologous or allogeneic stem cells from the bone marrow, peripheral blood, or cord blood, as described in chapter 6.

Screening for High-Risk Cancer-Causing Conditions. Cancer is more common in adults with certain syndromes or preexisting conditions. Screening allows early diagnosis with a better chance of cure. High-risk predisposing conditions exist for almost every type of cancer: (1) nonmelanoma skin cancer: Gorlin and nevoid basal cell carcinoma syndromes, immunosuppression, previous radiation, ultraviolet light exposure, arsenic psoriasis therapy; (2) prostate cancer: African Americans, family history; (3) breast cancer: *BRCA1* or *BRCA2* gene mutations, Li-Fraumeni (*p53* gene mutation), Cowden, Peutz-Jeghers, and Muir-Torre syndromes; (4) lung cancer: heavy smoking; (5) colon cancer: Gardner, Peutz-Jeghers, Turcot, familial polyposis (*APC* gene mutation), and hereditary nonpolyposis colorectal cancer (HNPCC) syndromes, previous radiation, inflammatory bowel disease; (6) uterine cancer: chronic estrogen therapy, obesity, diabetes mellitus, hypertension; (7) lymphoma: ataxia-telangietasia, neurofibromatosis type 1, and Li-Fraumeni syndromes, HIV infection; (8) bladder cancer: previous Cytoxan therapy, schistosoma infection; (9) ovarian cancer: *BRCA1* or *BRCA2* gene mutations, hereditary breast-ovarian cancer and HNPCC syndromes; (10) malignant melanoma: dysplastic-nevi, familial-atypical-multiple-mole-melanoma and xeroderma pigmentosa syndromes, retinoblastoma, previous radiation, ultraviolet light exposure, immunosuppression; (11) anorectal cancer: as for colon cancer; (12) oropharyngeal cancer: ataxia-telangietasia, Fanconi, and xeroderma pigmentosa syndromes; (13) leukemia: Downs, Li-Fraumeni, ataxia-telangietasia, Blooms, and Fanconi syndromes; (14) renal cancer: von Hippel-Lindau and familial papillary and clear cell carcinoma and oncocytoma syndromes; (15) pancreatic cancer: multiple endocrine neoplasia type 1, von Hippel-Lindau, ataxia-telangietasia, familial pancreatic cancer, and HNPCC syndromes, diabetes mellitus, chronic pancreatitis; (16) cervix cancer: immunosuppression, papilloma virus, and HIV infections; (17) stomach cancer: HNPCC, Li-Fraumeni, and familial gastric cancer syndromes, mucosa damage from previous radiation, pernicious anemia, gastric ulcer, chronic atrophic gastritis, *Helicobacter pylori* and Epstein-Barr virus infections; (18) brain tumor: Downs, Li-Fraumeni, ataxia-telangietasia, Gorlin, and neurofibromatosis type 1 syndromes, retinoblastoma, previous radiation; (19) liver and biliary tract cancer: Wilson disease, hemochromatosis, hereditary tyrosinemia, glycogen storage type 1, hepatic porphyria, familial polyposis coli, ataxia-telangietasia, neurofibromatosis, Budd-Chiari, and α-antitrypsin deficiency syndromes, hepatitis B and C, biliary atresia, cirrhosis, chemical carcinogens, fungal aflatoxin, alcohol, previous radiation; (20) multiple myeloma: family history, previous radiation, chemical carcinogens, alcohol, tobacco, herpes virus-8 infection, Kaposi sarcoma; (21) esophageal cancer: mucosa damage from strong tea, caustics, iron deficiency, previous radiation, Barrett's esophagus (chronic esophagitis), *Helicobacter pylori* and papilloma virus infections; (22) soft tissue sarcoma: Li-Fraumeni and Beckwith-Wiedemann syndromes, retinoblastoma, previous radiation; (23) testicular cancer: Klinefelter syndrome, undescended testes, genito-urinary anomalies, estrogen therapy during pregnancy; and (24) bone sarcoma: Li-Fraumeni syndrome, retinoblastoma, previous radiation.

9. Search for Cures

No single panacea will ever be able to cure all cancers, but the search for cures for each type of cancer has produced some remarkable discoveries. This chapter describes the principles underlying many promising novel therapies, some already in use, others still in the developmental stage. Such novel therapies include molecular targeted therapy, gene therapy, differentiating therapy, antiangiogenic therapy, antimetastatic therapy, multidrug resistance-reversal therapy, and preventive therapy. Since the endpoint of laboratory research is the application to patients, the clinical trial process will also be described.

Molecular Targeted Therapy

Principles Underlying Molecular Targeted Therapy.
Molecular targeted therapy, also called molecular therapy, involves blocking signaling pathways used by cells to sense the environment and communicate with each other. Such pathways regulate all aspects of cell functions, including division, maturation, repair, senescence, and apoptosis. Signal messages secreted by cells are called ligands or first messengers, and detectors of signals are called receptors. When ligands react with their receptors, they switch on other pathways and release small molecules, the second messengers, to further spread the signals. In normal cells, checks and balances regulate the signaling pathways. These checks and balances have become defective in cancer cells, allowing their escape from programs that control normal cells.

Molecular Therapy Targeting Vital Activities.   Some types of molecular therapy have been designed to act on vital activities such as DNA, RNA, protein synthesis, cell cycle checkpoints, senescence, and apoptosis by specifically targeting differences between cancer cells and normal cells.

Targeting DNA, RNA, and Protein Synthesis.   Normal DNA, RNA, and protein synthesis are described in chapter 3. In cancer cells the signaling pathways that regulate these functions may be defective, allowing endless DNA, RNA, and protein to be made for continuous cell division. Molecular therapy has been designed to correct such defective signaling pathways.

Targeting Cell Cycle Checkpoints.   Normal cell cycle checkpoints that control cells going through the cell cycle have been described in chapter 3. Some checkpoints regulate cell maturation or aging, while others allow damaged DNA to be repaired or the cells to be destroyed by apoptosis. In cancer cells, the signaling pathways that regulate these checkpoints may be defective, allowing cancer cells to continuously stay in the cell cycle and multiply relentlessly. Molecular therapy has been designed to correct such defective signaling pathways that had rendered the checkpoints nonfunctional.

Targeting Senescence.   During normal aging of cells, DNA is lost from the ends of the chromosomes that get shorter and shorter until the cells can no longer divide. To remedy this DNA loss, a special DNA polymerase enzyme, telomerase, is used to make a special type of DNA. Telomere DNA consists of six repeating nucleotides, TTAGGG, that are assembled on an RNA template instead of a DNA template, in a process called reverse transcription. In normal cells telomerase is switched off with maturation, so that telomere DNA is lost and the normal cells age and die. In cancer cells telomerase is not switched off, allowing endless DNA synthesis and cell division, and the cancer cells escape aging and death. Molecular therapy has been designed to "turn off" the high telomerase activity that confers virtual immortality to cancer cells.

Targeting Apoptosis. Signaling pathways also regulate the normal process of death of cells. A family of death enzymes, the caspases, are switched on to kill cells destined to die. A family of proapoptosis genes and proteins, the *BAX* family, promotes cell death, but another family of antiapoptosis genes and proteins, the *BCL-2* family, blocks cell death. Other oncogenes and tumor suppressor genes also play a role in regulating cell death. In cancer cells, the apoptosis pathways are defective, allowing their escape from the normal process of cell death. Molecular therapy has been designed to correct these defective apoptosis pathways that allow cancer cells to live on and accumulate relentlessly.

Molecular Therapy Targeting Essential Receptors. Other types of molecular therapy have been designed to act on essential receptors such as the tyrosine kinases, growth factor receptors, and G-proteins by specifically targeting additional differences between cancer cells and normal cells.

Blocking Tyrosine Kinases. Tyrosine kinases are enzymes that make up the most important receptors for processing signals. These receptors, which bridge the cell membranes, contain a pair of ligand-binding sites outside the cells and a pair of tyrosine kinase sites inside the cells. Their main function is to transmit signals from the outside of cells to within cells. Tyrosine kinase receptors are switched on by the substitution of a phosphate group for a hydroxyl group (phosphorylation), but switched off by the removal of a phosphate group (dephosphorylation).

Anticancer Opportunities. The best example of blocking a tyrosine kinase enzyme is the use of molecular therapy for treatment of chronic myelogenous leukemia, which carries a mutation called the "Philadelphia chromosome." This mutation, a mutual exchange of genetic material between the long arms of chromosomes 9 and 22 (reciprocal translocation), produces a fused oncogene (*ABL-BCR*) that makes a tyrosine kinase protein, p210. The energy source of the p210 protein is its adenosine triphosphate (ATP)-pocket, which has binding sites for ATP and other substances that react with p210. The p210 protein may be inactivated by blocking these binding sites with molecular therapy agents, including small peptides (short chains of amino acids), small-molecule inhibitors, and "mimic molecules." Mimic molecules are designed with five ligand arms to simultaneously block five different binding sites within the ATP-pocket. Alternatively, antisense oligonucleotides, short pieces of DNA that block mRNA from directing protein production, may be used to prevent the production of the p210 protein. The ABL kinase enzyme may also be blocked with inhibitors such as imatinib (Gleevec), dasatinib (Sprycel), and nilotinib (Tasigna).

Blocking Growth Factor Receptors.   Growth factor receptors are also tyrosine kinase enzymes. Growth factors are stimulants of cancer growth that may be targeted with molecular therapy. The best example is the HER2/neu receptor of breast carcinoma, which can be blocked with an anti-HER2/neu antibody, trastuzumab (Herceptin). Another example is the epidermal growth factor receptor (EGFR) present in many types of carcinomas, which can be blocked with antibodies (cetuximab, panitumumab), inhibitors (gefitinib/Iressa, erlotinib/Tarceva), or small molecules.

Blocking G-proteins.   G-proteins are another type of receptor. G-proteins are so-called because they contain a guanosine triphosphate (GTP)-pocket, similar to the ATP-pocket of tyrosine kinase receptors. The GTP-pocket has binding sites for GTP. The most important G-protein is the RAS protein made by *RAS* oncogene. The RAS protein is a vitally important receptor in many signaling pathways for activating transcription factors, which are substances that signal DNA to make RNA and protein. The RAS protein, which is normally bound to guanosine diphosphate (GDP), can be switched on by the addition of a phosphate group to make GTP, or switched off by the removal of a phosphate group to restore GDP.

Anticancer Opportunities.   The best example of blocking a G-protein is the use of molecular therapy for treatment of chronic myelogenous leukemia, melanoma, and gastrointestinal cancer, all of which express the RAS protein. Blocking binding sites in the GTP-pocket of the RAS protein with molecular therapy agents, such as small-molecule inhibitors and mimic molecules, inactivates the RAS protein. Alternatively, farnesyl transferase inhibitors may be used to block the farnesyl transferase enzyme that has the function of activating the RAS protein.

Gene Therapy

Gene Therapy with Target Genes.   Gene therapy treats cancer by introducing target genes that can boost immunity, kill tumor cells, or protect the bone marrow from chemotherapy. Carriers that put target genes into cells are called vectors. Vectors are usually RNA retroviruses. Gene therapy is similar to some aspects of natural viral infections in which viruses enter human cells, use their reverse transcriptase enzyme to make viral DNA from viral mRNA, integrate the viral DNA into human DNA, and use the human DNA machinery to multiply and package viruses for release to infect other human cells. In gene therapy, retroviral vectors are used that have intact packaging instructions but do not contain the structural protein genes necessary for multiplying within human cells. Target genes are put into the retroviral vectors. These retroviral vectors are then inserted into packaging cells. Viral structural protein genes necessary for multiplying are also inserted into the packaging cells, but at locations separate from the retroviral vectors. The packaging cells can then package and release the multiplied retroviral vectors containing target genes to infect cancer cells. However, the packaging cells cannot package or release the viral structural protein genes, which lack packaging instructions, to infect normal cells.

Gene Therapy for Boosting Immunity. Gene therapy may be used boost immunity to help patients fight their cancers. One example is inserting genes that produce natural immune substances involved in the killing of cancer cells (e.g., interleukins, tumor necrosis factor, interferons) into certain lymphocytes (e.g., killer T cells, natural killer cells, tumor-infiltrating lymphocytes) to enhance their ability to kill cancer cells. Another example is inserting tumor antigens into viruses or into cells that have long cytoplasmic processes for capturing and presenting antigens (dendritic cells), to make vaccines for immunizing patients against their own cancers. A third example is to treat patients with donor cancer-killing T cells that have been preprogrammed for destruction once their mission is accomplished, by inserting a herpes simplex virus "suicide gene" that make them susceptible to antiviral therapy.

Gene Therapy for Killing Cancer Cells. Gene therapy may be used to stop the excessive proliferation of cancer cells, by restoring the regulatory function of tumor suppressor genes or by blocking the stimulatory activity of oncogenes. One example is inserting a normal *p53* tumor suppressor gene to restore the loss of control caused by a *p53* mutation in cancer cells. Another example is inserting antisense oligonucleotides, which are short pieces of DNA that block mRNA from directing protein production, to prevent the excessive production MYC protein caused by a *MYC* oncogene mutation in cancer cells. A third example is to use RNA enzymes (ribozymes) to break up mRNA and suppress RAS protein production caused by a *RAS* oncogene mutation in cancer cells. A fourth example is injecting herpes simplex virus "suicide genes" into brain tumor cells, and then using antiviral therapy to kill both the viruses and the brain tumor cells.

Gene Therapy for Targeting Viruses. Gene therapy may be used to modify viruses so that they can replicate only in cancer cells. One example is making an adenovirus that lacks a certain protein, the E1B protein, so that it cannot replicate in normal cells that can produce p53 protein. The function of the p53 protein is to trigger the death of infected cells, so as to prevent viral infection from spreading. Many types of cancer cells contain *p53* mutations so that they cannot produce p53 protein. The E1B-defective adenovirus inserted by gene therapy will only replicate in and kill the cancer cells containing *p53* mutations that cannot make p53 protein.

Gene Therapy for Protecting Bone Marrow from Chemotherapy. Gene therapy may be used to protect the bone marrow in patients undergoing high-dose chemotherapy for breast cancer or bone marrow transplant. One example is inserting a *MDR1* gene into bone marrow cells to make them resistant to the toxic effects of chemotherapy. The *MDR1* gene directs the production of P-glycoprotein, which acts as a "pump" to remove natural-product drugs from cancer cells, making them resistant to chemotherapy, as described in chapter 3.

Gene Therapy for Targeting DNA Tumor Viruses. Gene therapy may be used to destroy certain DNA tumor viruses that can initiate many types of cancers. Examples include the human papilloma virus (HPV) that causes cervix carcinoma and the Epstein-Barr virus (EBV) that causes lymphoma and AIDS-related cancers. These DNA tumor viruses also produce proteins that can stimulate tumor growth. Antisense oligonucleotides may be used to block the function of HPV and EBV mRNA. Alternatively, inhibitors may be used to block the DNA-binding sites or other contact regions for HPV and EBV.

Differentiating Therapy

Underlying Principle. Cancer cells retain the ability to replicate relentlessly because they have not undergone differentiation. Differentiating therapy treats cancer by inducing maturation of cancer cells with compounds such as vitamin A derivatives (retinoids), vitamin D derivatives, and inhibitors of the histone deacetylase enzyme.

Retinoids. Retinoids are compounds that can stop cell division, cause differentiation, and prevent cancers from starting. Retinoids must be activated by binding first to the retinoic acid receptor and then to the retinoid X receptor. The activated retinoids then act on target genes, regulating the DNA that directs the production of mRNA and proteins.

Anticancer Opportunities. Different retinoids may be used as differentiating agents for treating different types of leukemia and cancer. One example is the treatment of acute promyelocytic leukemia, which contains a mutation in which there is a mutual exchange of genetic material between the long arms of chromosomes 15 and 17 (reciprocal translocation). This mutation produces a fused cancer gene, which makes a protein that can be blocked by all-*trans*-retinoic acid (ATRA), or by arsenic trioxide. Another example is using 13-*cis*-retinoic acid for differentiation of myelodysplastic syndrome (a blood disorder that often develops into leukemia), chronic myelogenous leukemia, germ cell tumors, cutaneous T-cell lymphoma, neuroblastoma, and skin cancer. A third example is using 9-*cis*-retinoic acid for differentiation of acute promyelocytic leukemia and AIDS-related Kaposi sarcoma. Retinoids have also been used to prevent head-and-neck, airway, and gastrointestinal cancers.

Vitamin D Compounds.   The active agent 1,25-dihydroxy-vitamin D_3 has been used for differentiation of bone marrow cells in myelodysplastic syndrome.

Differentiating Agents Working Through the Coiling and Uncoiling of DNA.   Normally, the DNA within chromosomes is coiled tightly around proteins called histones. Before transcription factors can bind to the DNA to direct the production of mRNA and proteins, the tightly coiled DNA must first unwind. The uncoiling of DNA is caused by the removal of a methyl group (demethylation) together with the addition of an acetyl group (histone acetylation). Conversely, the uncoiling of DNA is prevented by the addition of a methyl group (methylation) together with the removal of an acetyl group (histone deacetylation).

Anticancer Opportunities.   Differentiating agents working through the coiling and uncoiling of DNA that may be used for treating myelodysplastic syndrome include azacytidine, a DNA demethylating agent, and trichostatin A, a histone deacetylation inhibitor. Another example is using sodium phenylbutyrate, a histone acetylating agent, for differentiation of acute promyelocytic leukemia.

Antiangiogenic Therapy

Neoplastic Angiogenesis.   Neoplastic angiogenesis is the laying down of new blood vessels by tumors. Those blood vessels provide the oxygen and nutrients necessary for growth. Cancers can produce their own proangiogenic factors to promote blood vessel growth, while immune cells infiltrating cancers can produce antiangiogenic factors to block blood vessel growth. Many stimuli, such as low oxygen, acidity, cytokines, growth factors, oncogenes, and tumor suppressor genes, interact to regulate neoplastic angiogenesis. These stimuli control the growth, survival and death of blood vessel and capillary cells, the production and binding of angiogenic factors to receptors on the blood vessels, and the migration, invasion, and spread of cancer cells. There are many natural proangiogenic factors, but the most important one is vascular endothelial growth factor (VEGF). There are also many natural antiangiogenic factors, but the main ones are transforming growth factor-β and tumor necrosis factor-α. In addition, many other growth factors, cytokines, and immune substances can also support or inhibit neoplastic angiogenesis.

Anticancer Opportunities. Antiangiogenic therapy uses molecular therapy for preventing neoplastic angiogenesis and destroying cancers. It may work by inhibiting natural proangiogenic factors, enhancing the effects of natural antiangiogenic factors or blocking angiogenic receptors on blood vessels.

Inhibiting Proangiogenic Activity. Agents such as thalidomide, endostatin, and angiostatin have been used as inhibitors to stop the growth of blood vessel cells. Antibodies against VEGF, such as bevacizumab (Avastin), and antibodies against the VEGF receptor have been used to block the activities of VEGF and other proangiogenic factors.

Enhancing Antiangiogenic Activity. Cytokines, such as interleukins and interferons, have antiangiogenic activity. The nonsteroidal anti-inflammatory drugs (NSAIDs) that are cyclooxygenase-2 (COX-2) enzyme inhibitors, celecoxib (Celebrex) and rofecoxib (Vioxx), also have antiangiogenic activity but are presently under investigation for possibly increasing the risk of heart attacks. Low-dose chemotherapy drugs, such as vinblastine, vincristine, or etoposide, have antiangiogenic activity, and may be used in combination with antibodies against VEGF and its receptor.

Blocking Angiogenic Receptors on Blood Vessels. Small-molecule inhibitors or chimeric immunoconjugates have been used to block angiogenic receptors on blood vessels. Chimeric immunoconjugates are molecules made by fusing parts of antiangiogenic antibodies and blood vessel receptors.

Antimetastatic Therapy

The Metastatic Process. The metastatic process is how cancer cells migrate, invade, and spread. These cancer cells detach from the main tumor, invade into lymphatics, small veins and capillaries, and stick to each other, to platelets, and to lymphocytes to form tumor clumps. As the tumor clumps move through the blood vessels, they become trapped in capillaries, stick to the capillary walls (adherence), invading through the capillary walls to spread into tissues and organs as metastases. The metastatic process depends on the movements of cancer cells, their sticking to each other and to capillary walls, their invading through tissues, and their settling in suitable environments and acquiring tumor blood supplies to support the growth of metastases. These functions depend on molecules on the cell surface (e.g., integrins, cadherins, CD44 glycoprotein, immunoglobulins), and certain enzymes (metalloproteinases, plasminogen). Integrins sense the environment and signal cancer cells to coordinate their movement, adherence, and invasiveness. Cadherins, CD44, and immunoglobulins allow cancer cells to stick to each other and to capillary walls.

Metalloproteinases dissolve the basement membranes of blood vessel cells, allowing cancer cells to invade into small blood vessels and break down tissue barriers.

Anticancer Opportunities.   Antimetastatic therapy treats cancer by inhibiting the metastatic process. One example is to use metalloproteinase inhibitors, such as Marimastat and Neovastat, to block the enzymes that help cancer cells invade blood vessels and break down tissue barriers during the metastatic process. Another example is to use the calcium-related angiogenesis inhibitor (CAI) to block cadherins that allow cancer cells to stick to each other and to capillary walls. A third example is to use small-molecule inhibitors and small peptides that mimic integrins, blocking the integrin receptors and preventing the spread of cancer.

Multidrug Resistance-reversal Therapy

Multidrug Resistance.   Drug resistance is a change in cancer cells so that they cannot be killed by drugs. Multidrug resistance is an adaptation of cancer cells that makes them resistant to several classes of drugs, and is one of the biggest problems during chemotherapy. The most important form of multidrug resistance is caused by mutation of the *MDR1* gene, or increased production of its protein, the P-glycoprotein. The *MDR1* gene has been preserved through evolution because it is a protective mechanism in the body against toxins in the environment. P-glycoprotein is naturally found in intestinal, kidney, and liver cells, bone marrow, and blood vessel cells, and forms protective barriers for the brain (blood-brain barrier), eye (blood-eye barrier), and testes (blood-testicular barrier). P-glycoprotein is a "drug pump" that can eliminate many classes of drugs that are natural products of plants and fungi, such as the vinca alkaloids (vincristine, vinblastine, vindesine) from the periwinkle plant, podophyllotoxins (etoposide, teniposide) from mandrake root and May apple, antibiotics (doxorubicin, daunorubicin, idarubicin, epirubicin, mitoxantrone, dactinomycin) from *Streptomyces* fungal species, and taxanes (Taxol, docetaxel) from Pacific yew tree bark. In many types of malignancies, the production of P-glycoprotein has been increased. These malignancies include leukemia, lymphoma, multiple myeloma, neuroblastoma, osteosarcoma, rhabdomyosarcoma, retinoblastoma, and many types of carcinomas. Chemotherapy cannot successfully cure these malignancies. As described in chapter 3, there are also less common causes of multidrug resistance, such as the multidrug resistance protein (MRP), breast cancer resistance protein (BCRP), lung resistance protein (LRP), topoisomerase II enzyme, and the glutathione family of enzymes, but it is still uncertain whether these entities cause a major problem in the clinic. Multidrug resistance-reversal therapy is the prevention of resistance to drugs used for treatment of cancer, and at present is available only for targeting P-glycoprotein.

Multidrug Resistance-Reversal Therapy Targeting P-glycoprotein. In general terms, the function of P-glycoprotein in cancer cells may be blocked at several levels. Therapy may be aimed at blocking the *MDR1* gene to stop *MDR1* mRNA from being made; inhibiting *MDR1* mRNA to stop P-glycoprotein from being made; or inactivating P-glycoprotein itself by inhibiting P-glycoprotein's function, blocking its drug pump activity, making drugs less susceptible to the effects of P-glycoprotein, and enhancing the killing of cancer cells. Alternatively, therapy may be aimed at enhancing the function of P-glycoprotein in normal cells, enabling them to better withstand the toxic effects of chemotherapy. One major disadvantage of multidrug resistance-reversal therapy is its associated increase in chemotherapy toxicity, because any therapy that can block P-glycoprotein in cancer cells will also inhibit its important protective function in normal intestinal, kidney, and liver cells, bone marrow, and blood vessel cells.

Blocking MDR1 Gene Function. The ability of the *MDR1* gene to signal mRNA production may be targeted. One example is to block the *MDR1* gene at its mRNA production start-site (promoter region) by using chemicals to link together and damage the two DNA strands. A second example is using short chains of DNA (DNA oligomers) to block the front part of the *MDR1* gene. A third example is using all-*trans* retinoid acid with dimethyl sulfoxide to differentiate the *MDR1* gene, so that it will not function properly. A fourth example is inhibiting DNA with drugs (e.g., 8-Cl-cAMP), so that *MDR1* mRNA cannot be made. A fifth example is using anti-sense mRNA, which are short pieces of RNA, to block the *MDR1* gene from directing the transcription of *MDR1* mRNA.

Inhibiting MDR1 mRNA Function. The ability of the MDR1 mRNA to direct P-glycoprotein production may be targeted. One example is inhibiting mRNA activity by using RNA enzymes (ribozymes) to break up the *MDR1* mRNA. A second example is inhibiting the function of *MDR1* mRNA with drugs such as mitomycin C or cisplatin. A third example is using antisense oligonucleotides, which are short pieces of DNA, to block *MDR1* mRNA and prevent the making of P-glycoprotein.

Inactivating P-glycoprotein Function. There are a number of inhibitors of P-glycoprotein, which compete with the pumping of drugs out of cancer cells. Verapamil is one such inhibitor, but it has been found to be too toxic to the heart. The amido-keto pipecolinate derivative VX-710 is another such inhibitor. The most commonly used inhibitor is cyclo-sporine A, or other cyclosporin derivatives such as PSC 833. Cyclosporins work mainly by inhibiting P-glycoprotein, but can also enhance the entry of drugs into the central nervous system and the eye, and improve the actions of carboplatin and etoposide by alternative mechanisms. However, blocking the P-glycoprotein in cancers cells with cyclosporins can also concurrently inhibit the P-glycoprotein protective mechanism in normal cells, producing more toxicity to chemotherapy. Furthermore, cyclosporins also slow down the breaking up and excretion of chemotherapy from the body by the kidneys and liver. Therefore, increased toxicity from chemotherapy has been found in many such clinical trials for multiple myeloma, lymphoma, acute myelogenous leukemia, osteosar-coma, and carcinomas. Only in clinical trials for retinoblas-toma, which uniquely give short infusions of cyclosporine A over hours rather than over days, has the improved effective-ness of chemotherapy not been offset by the increased toxicity from chemotherapy.

Inactivating P-glycoprotein "Drug Pump" Activity. Anti-bodies against P-glycoprotein (e.g., MRK16, HYB241) have been made to block the function of the P-glycoprotein drug pump. Such antibodies may also be used together with cyclosporine A for greater effectiveness.

Making Drugs Less Susceptible to the Effects of P-glycoprotein. Drugs may be altered in some way to make them less susceptible to the effects of P-glycoprotein. One exam-ple is changing doxorubicin into its 9-alkyl morpholinyl derivative, which is less susceptible to the effects of P-glycoprotein. A second example is packaging doxorubicin into lipid cap-sules (liposomes) for better delivery into cancer cells. A third example is using certain peptides (e.g., defensin, cecropin), or packaging with a P-glycoprotein inhibitor (e.g., cyclosporine A), to make doxorubicin more potent for killing cancer cells.

Enhancing the Killing of Cancer Cells.   Combination therapy with two or more killing agents may be used to enhance the cancer cell kill. One example is combining a toxin (e.g., *Pseudomonas* bacterial toxin, ricin poison) with an inhibitor of P-glycoprotein (e.g., antibody against P-glycoprotein, chemotherapy-antibody combination).

Enhancing P-glycoprotein Function in Normal Cells to Better Withstand Chemotherapy Toxicity.   This may be achieved by gene therapy. An example is inserting the *MDR1* gene into bone marrow cells, protecting them from toxicity during high-dose chemotherapy for breast cancer and bone marrow transplant.

Preventive Therapy

Underlying Principles.   Preventive therapy introduces natural products, dietary supplements, or drugs to prevent the recurrence of cancer or the development of secondary cancers caused by radiation. Preventive therapy also means avoiding known carcinogens such as sunlight that can cause skin cancer, tobacco that can cause lung cancer, and toxins of fungi contaminating food that can cause liver cancer. It additionally means avoiding certain factors, such as excess fat in the diet, that may increase the risk of breast, colon, uterus, prostate, and other cancers. Preventive therapy, however, cannot cure established cancers. Furthermore, measuring the benefit from preventive therapy is very difficult, since the reduction of cancer risk may be small. To prove that preventive therapy really is beneficial, huge clinical trials have to be done that give the treatment over many years.

Anticancer Opportunities.   Many compounds are reported to have cancer-preventing properties. Vegetables, fruits, beans, and nuts are thought to prevent cancer because of their carotenoid, phytoestrogen, organosulfur, organoselenium, and protease inhibitor contents. High-fiber diets are thought to prevent colorectal, breast, and other cancers. The vitamin A derivatives, retinoids and carotenoids, are thought to prevent cancer. Retinoids have differentiating properties, and carotenoids in green and yellow fruits and vegetables are natural antioxidants that break down carcinogens and cause differentiation. These vitamin A derivatives have been used to treat premalignant lesions in the mouth, lung, skin, and cervix, as well as head-and-neck, breast, and bladder cancers. Calcium supplement has been used in colorectal cancer trials. Selenium, a micronutrient, has been used in skin, colorectal, lung, and prostate cancer trials. Some cancer-preventing trials have combined a number of multivitamins and micronutrients, including carotenoids, vitamin C, and vitamin E. Other cancer-preventing trials have used aspirin or nonsteroidal anti-inflammatory drugs (NSAIDs) in patients with the familial adenomatous polyposis syndrome, in which multiple polyps can develop into colorectal cancer. Presently, the NSAIDs celecoxib (Celebrex) and rofecoxib (Vioxx) are under investigation for possibly increasing the risk of heart attacks.

New Drug Development and the Clinical Trial Process

New Drug Development.   Development of new drugs goes through many stages before they reach the clinic. First, drugs are screened for effectiveness using cancer cell lines in the laboratory. They are then tested for their absorption, breakdown,

Table 9.1 Summary of Novel Therapies and How They Work

Classes	Mechanisms of Action	Drugs and Agents	Diseases Treated
Molecular targeted therapy	blocking tyrosine kinase receptors	(1) small peptides (2) small-molecule inhibitors (3) p210 protein ATP-pocket "mimic molecules" (4) antisense oligonucleotides	Philadelphia chromosome-positive chronic myelogenous leukemia with a fused oncogene producing p210 protein
	blocking growth factor receptors	(1) anti-HER2/neu antibody trastuzumab (Herceptin) (2) small-molecule inhibitors	HER2/neu receptor-positive breast carcinoma
		(1) anti-EGFR monoclonal antibody (2) small-molecule inhibitors	epidermal growth factor receptor (EGFR)-positive breast, stomach, esophagus, head-and-neck, ovarian, and lung carcinoma
	blocking RAS G-protein receptor	(1) small-molecule inhibitors (2) RAS protein GTP-pocket "mimic molecules" (3) farnesyl transferase inhibitors	RAS protein-expressing chronic myelogenous leukemia, melanoma, and gastrointestinal cancer
Gene therapy	boosting immunity	(1) inserting interleukin, interferon, or tumor necrosis factor genes into immune killer lymphocytes to enhance their ability to kill cancer cells	melanoma, sarcoma, chronic myelogenous leukemia, renal cell, prostate, and colorectal cancer

(Continued)

Table 9.1 (Continued)

Classes	Mechanisms of Action	Drugs and Agents	Diseases Treated
		(2) inserting tumor antigens into viruses or dendritic cells to make vaccines for immunizing patients against their own cancers	
		(3) using donor cancer-killing T cells with inserted herpes simplex virus "suicide gene" that allows destruction by antiviral therapy	
	killing cancer cells	(1) inserting a normal p53 tumor suppressor gene into cancer cells to restore the loss of control caused by p53 mutations	non-Hodgkin lymphoma, chronic myelogenous leukemia, brain tumor, mesothelioma, non–small cell lung, prostate, head-and-neck, ovarian, and colorectal cancer
		(2) antisense oligonucleotides to stop MYC protein production caused by a MYC oncogene mutation	
		(3) ribozymes to break up mRNA and suppress RAS protein production caused by a RAS oncogene mutation	
		(4) injecting herpes simplex virus "suicide genes" into brain tumor cells and then use antiviral therapy to kill both the viruses and the brain tumor cells	

	targeting viruses	inserting an E1B-defective adenovirus that replicates and kills cancer cells that produce no p53 protein due to $p53$ mutations	head-and-neck cancer
	protecting bone marrow from chemotherapy	inserting a $MDR1$ gene into bone marrow cells, to make them resistant to the toxic effects of high-dose chemotherapy	breast cancer, bone marrow transplant
	targeting DNA tumor viruses	(1) HPV antisense oligonucleotides to block mRNA from directing protein production	cervix carcinoma caused by human papilloma virus (HPV)
		(2) inhibitors of HPV DNA-binding sites or other contact regions	
		(1) EBV antisense oligonucleotides to block mRNA from directing protein production	lymphoma and AIDS-related cancers caused by Epstein-Barr virus (EBV)
		(2) inhibitors of EBV DNA-binding sites or other contact regions	
Differentiating therapy	retinoids	(1) all-*trans*-retinoic acid (ATRA)	acute promyelocytic leukemia
		(2) arsenic trioxide 13-*cis*-retinoic acid	myelodysplastic syndrome, chronic myelogenous leukemia, germ cell tumors, cutaneous T-cell lymphoma, skin cancer, neuroblastoma

(Continued)

Table 9.1 (*Continued*)

Classes	Mechanisms of Action	Drugs and Agents	Diseases Treated
	vitamin D compounds	9-*cis*-retinoic acid	acute promyelocytic leukemia and AIDS-related Kaposi sarcoma
		1,25-dihydroxyvitamin D_3	myelodysplastic syndrome
	differentiating agents working on DNA coiling and uncoiling	(1) azacytidine, a DNA demethylating agent (2) trichostatin A, a histone deacetylation inhibitor	myelodysplastic syndrome
		sodium phenylbutyrate, a histone acetylating agent	acute promyelocytic leukemia
Antiangiogenic therapy	inhibiting proangiogenic activity	(1) thalidomide, endostatin, angiostatin as inhibitors to stop growth of blood vessel cells	massive infantile hemangioma, giant cell tumor of mandible, Kaposi sarcoma, bladder and other cancers
		(2) antibodies against VEGF and its receptor for blocking the activities of VEGF and other proangiogenic factors	
	enhancing antiangiogenic activity	(1) cytokines such as interleukins and interferons	refractory to conventional chemotherapy
		(2) nonsteroidal anti-inflammatory drugs, celecoxib (Celebrex) and rofecoxib (Vioxx),	

		(3) low-dose vinblastine, vincristine, or etoposide chemotherapy; may be used with antibodies against VEGF and its receptor which are presently under investigation for possibly increasing the risk of heart attacks	
	blocking angiogenic receptors on blood vessels	(1) small-molecule inhibitors	melanoma
		(2) chimeric immunoconjugates made by fusing together parts of antiangiogenic antibodies and blood vessel receptors	
Antimetastatic therapy	blocking metalloproteinase enzymes	(1) metalloproteinase inhibitors, Marimastat and Neovastat, to block enzymes that help cancer cells invade into blood vessels and break down tissue barriers	cancers refractory to conventional chemotherapy
		(2) calcium-related angiogenic inhibitor (CAI), to block cadherins that allow cancer cells to stick to each other and to capillary walls	
	blocking cadherin	calcium-related angiogenesis inhibitor (CAI) blocks cadherins that allow cancer cells to stick to each other and to capillary walls	cancers refractory to conventional chemotherapy
	blocking integrin receptors	(1) small-molecule inhibitors	colon cancer
		(2) small peptides that mimic integrins	

(Continued)

Table 9.1 *(Continued)*

Classes	Mechanisms of Action	Drugs and Agents	Diseases Treated
Multidrug resistance-reversal therapy	blocking *MDR1* gene function	(1) blocking *MDR1* gene promoter region by chemical cross-linking the two DNA strands	not yet in clinical trials
		(2) DNA oligomers to block the front part of the *MDR1* gene	
		(3) all-*trans* retinoid acid with dimethyl sulfoxide to differentiate the *MDR1* gene	
		(4) inhibiting DNA with drugs (e.g., 8-Cl-cAMP) preventing *MDR1* mRNA production	
		(5) antisense mRNA to block *MDR1* mRNA transcription	
	inhibiting *MDR1* mRNA function	(1) RNA enzymes (ribozymes) to break up the *MDR1* mRNA	not yet in clinical trials
		(2) inhibiting the function of *MDR1* mRNA with drugs such as mitomycin C or cisplatin	
		(3) antisense oligonucleotides to block *MDR1* mRNA from making P-glycoprotein	
	inactivating P-glycoprotein function	(1) verapamil	clinical trials for multiple myeloma, lymphoma, acute
		(2) amido-keto pipecolinate derivative, VX-710	

Goal	Method	Status
inactivating P-glycoprotein "drug pump" activity	(3) cyclosporine A, or other cyclosporin derivatives such as PSC 833	myelogenous leukemia, osteosarcoma, carcinoma, brain tumor, and retinoblastoma
	(1) antibodies against P-glycoprotein (e.g., MRK16, HYB241)	not yet in clinical trials
	(2) antibodies against P-glycoprotein used in combination with cyclosporine A	
making drugs less susceptible to the effects of P-glycoprotein	(1) changing doxorubicin into its 9-alkyl morpholinyl derivative that is less susceptible to P-glycoprotein	not yet in clinical trials
	(2) packaging doxorubicin into liposomes for better delivery into cancer cells	
	(3) using defensin or cecropin peptides, or packaging with cyclosporine A, to make doxorubicin more potent for killing cancer cells	
enhancing the killing of cancer cells	combining a toxin (e.g., *Pseudomonas* bacterial toxin, ricin poison) with an inhibitor of P-glycoprotein (e.g., antibody against P-glycoprotein, chemotherapy-antibody combination)	not yet in clinical trials
enhancing P-glycoprotein	inserting the *MDR1* gene into bone marrow cells to protect them from chemotherapy	high-dose chemotherapy for breast cancer and bone marrow

(Continued)

Table 9.1 (*Continued*)

Classes	Mechanisms of Action	Drugs and Agents	Diseases Treated
	function in normal cells to better withstand chemotherapy toxicity	toxicity	transplant
Preventive therapy	avoiding carcinogens	(1) known carcinogens include sunlight, tobacco, and toxins of fungi (2) factors that may increase the risk of many types of cancer include excess fat in the diet	prevention of skin, lung, liver, breast, colon, uterus, prostate, and other cancers
	dietary anticarcinogens	carotenoids, phytoestrogens, organosulfur, organoselenium, and protease inhibitors in vegetables, fruits, beans, and nuts	cancer prevention in general
	high-fiber diet	bran, oat, vegetables, fruits	prevention of colorectal, breast, and other cancers
	vitamin A derivatives	retinoids, carotenoids in green and yellow fruits and vegetables	treatment of premalignant lesions in the mouth, lung, skin, and cervix, as well as head-and-neck, breast, and bladder cancers

calcium	calcium supplements	colorectal cancer
selenium	the micronutrient selenium	skin, colorectal, lung, and prostate cancers
multivitamins and micronutrients	carotenoids, vitamin C and vitamin E combinations	cancer-preventing trials
anti-inflammatory drugs	(1) aspirin (2) nonsteroidal anti-inflammatory drugs celecoxib (Celebrex) and rofecoxib (Vioxx), although presently under investigation for possibly increasing the risk of heart attacks	colorectal cancer-preventing trials in patients with familial adenomatous polyposis syndrome

and excretion in animals and their entry into the central nervous system. The best way to manufacture the drug is determined, and the best route for administration according to its absorption and distribution in animals. Testing of organ toxicity and safe starting dose are carried out in animals. The risks of inducing gene mutations (mutagenesis) and cancer (carcinogenesis) are tested in animals. The risk of inducing fetal damage during pregnancy (teratogenesis) is also tested in animals. After this, new drugs are tested in a series of clinical trials in human patients.

Phase I Clinical Trial.   The aims are to determine the tolerance to the drug and its pharmacology, rather than the anticancer effects in patients with all types of advanced cancer for which there is no conventional therapy.

Phase II Clinical Trial.   The aims are to determine the anticancer effects, dosages, and toxicity in patients with one particular type of advanced cancer for which there is no conventional therapy.

Phase III Clinical Trial.   The aims are to determine in a randomized, controlled trial the anticancer effects, dosages, and toxicity of a new drug (experimental arm), compared to the current standard drug (control arm). The patients all have to have the same type of cancer and be previously untreated. A randomized trial means that one half of the patients are randomly designated to receive the experimental arm, and the other half the control arm. A controlled trial means that the number of patients recruited (sample size) is calculated beforehand to make sure that the results can answer the questions of whether the experimental arm is more effective and less toxic than the control arm. In a controlled trial, patient characteristics (e.g., age range, stage of disease, favorable and unfavorable prognostic factors) also have to be similar for both the experimental arm and the control arm. For rare cancers in which patient numbers are too small for a randomized trial, the results of the new treatment may be compared with that of the previous treatment (historical controls).

Phase IV Clinical Trial. The aims are to determine in a randomized, controlled trial the anticancer effects and immediate (acute) and long-term (chronic) toxicities of a new regimen combining chemotherapy, surgery, radiation, and/or new therapies (experimental arm), compared to the current standard regimen (control arm). The patients all have to have the same type of cancer and be previously untreated.

Regulation of Clinical Trials. Clinical trials are now heavily regulated from ethical and safety standpoints, to protect patients and make sure that the results are accurate and collected properly. Regulators of clinical trials include internal scientific reviews, institutional review boards (IRBs), and governmental regulatory agencies (Food and Drug Administration and National Cancer Institute/National Institutes of Health in the United States, and Health Canada in Canada). Consent forms are required, which clearly explain in simple language the potential benefits of the treatment and possible risks of complications (risk-benefit ratio), and any alternative therapy options. This is for the protection of the patients and their families, making sure that they have all the information necessary for decision making. In summary, the goal of each clinical trial is to establish new "gold standards" for treating a particular type of cancer, improving on both the effectiveness and toxicity of the previous standard treatment.

Appendix

Internet resources

Main cancer agencies websites. The educated consumer of today's world usually searches the Internet for further information when he/she or a family member is diagnosed with cancer. There are websites for specific types of cancers, such as leukemia, lymphoma, multiple myeloma, brain tumor, and breast, prostate, lung, eye, genitourinary, gastrointestinal, head-and-neck, and skin cancer. There are also websites for pediatric malignancies, bone marrow transplant, and on statistics, genetics, prevention, treatment, and literature on cancer. Some general websites are listed below. A more extensive list may be accessed through the National Cancer Institute website. There are links to specific disease websites, and to major U.S., Canadian, and European cancer organizations.

Research and treatment centers. A list of cancer research and treatment centers in the U.S. (NCI Cancer Center Websites) and Europe (Sustaining Oncology Studies Europe) can be accessed through the Internet.

Cancer literature websites. Cancer literature and disease summaries are now available online, but the articles are usually directed to health professionals.

Treatment cooperative groups. Childhood and adult cancers are now generally treated under the auspices of a cooperative group, on clinical trials or standard protocols. For example, childhood cancer treatment is standardized through the Children's Oncology Group (COG). In Europe, the equivalent is the International Society of Pediatric Oncology (SIOP). In the U.S., major cooperative groups for adult cancer treatment include the Southwest Oncology Group (SWOG), Eastern Cooperative Oncology Group (ECOG), and American College of Surgeons Oncology Group (ACOSOG). In Europe, there is the European Organization for Research and Treatment of Cancer (EORTC).

Professional associations for cancer research and treatment. These websites are usually accessible only by health professionals, members of the associations.

Family support groups. All cancer centers have family support groups. National and international support groups can also be accessed through the Internet.

Internet Resources for Cancer

General national and international cancer agencies

National Cancer Institute (USA)
http://nci.nih.gov

National Cancer Institute of Canada
www.ncic.cancer.ca

Specialized cancer websites with links to specific disease websites

American Cancer Society
http://www.cancer.org

Canadian Cancer Society
http://www.cancer.ca

Cancer Education
http://www.cancereducation.com

National Cancer Institute Cancer Information Service
http://cis.nci.nih.gov

CDC National Program of Cancer Registries
http://www.cdc.gov/cancer/npcr

Registered clinical trials
http://www.clinicaltrials.gov

Research and treatment centers

National Cancer Institute Cancer Center Websites
http://www.nci.nih.gov/cancercenters/centerslist.html

Sustaining Oncology Studies Europe
http://sos.unige.it/soseuro.html

Cancer literature websites

MEDLINE*plus*
http://www.nlm.nih.gov/medlineplus/cancers.html

OncoLink
http://oncolink.upenn.edu

CancerLit
http://www.cancer.gov/search/cancer_literature

Physician Data Query (PDQ) adult and childhood cancer
summaries
http://www.cancer.gov/cancertopics/pdq

EMedicine Journal disease summaries
http://www.eMedicine.com

Cancer treatment cooperative groups

Children's Oncology Group
http://www.childrensoncologygroup.org

International Society of Pediatric Oncology (SIOP)
http://www.siop.nl

Southwest Oncology Group (SWOG)
http://www.swog.org

Eastern Cooperative Oncology Group (ECOG)
http://ecog.dfci.harvard.edu

American College of Surgeons Oncology Group
(ACOSOG)
https://www.acosog.org

European Organization for Research and Treatment of
Cancer (EORTC)
http://www.eortc.be

International Union Against Cancer (UICC)
http://www.uicc.org

Professional associations for cancer research and treatment

American Association for Cancer Research
http://www.aacr.org

American Society for Clinical Oncology
http://www.asco.org

Oncology Nursing Society
http://www.ons.org

Society of Surgical Oncology
http://www.surgonc.org

Family support groups

Association of Cancer Online Resources
http://www.acor.org/index.html

Candlelighters Childhood Cancer Foundation
http://www.candlelighters.org

Outlook: Life Beyond Childhood Cancer
http://www.outlook-life.org

Make-A-Wish Foundation of America
http://www.wish.org

The Children's Wish Foundation of Canada
http://www.childrenswish.ca

Ronald McDonald House Charities
http://www.rmhc.com

Index

Understanding Health and Sickness Series
Miriam Bloom, Ph.D., General Editor

Also in this series

Addiction • Alzheimer's Disease • Anemia • Asthma • Breast Cancer
Genetics • Child Sexual Abuse • Childhood Obesity • Chronic Pain •
Colon Cancer • Cosmetic Laser Surgery • Crohn Disease and
Ulcerative Colitis • Cystic Fibrosis • Dental Health • Depression •
Hepatitis • Herpes • Mental Retardation • Migraine and Other
Headaches • Multiple Sclerosis • Panic and Other Anxiety Disorders •
Sickle Cell Disease • Stuttering